Empowering Women to Embrace Menopause with Confidence

Navigating the Power Shift in Women's Lives, and the Liberation of Midlife: A Guide to Empowering Change and Embracing Wellness for Women

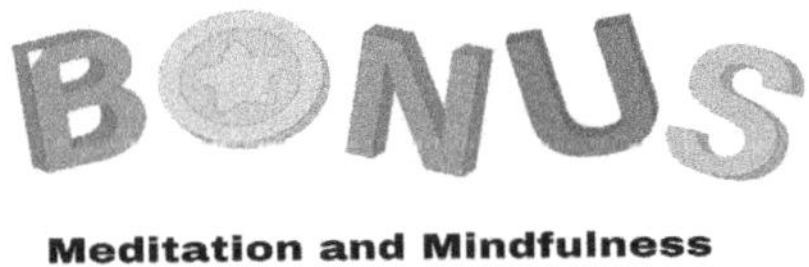

Meditation and Mindfulness

Teresa M. Broaddus

Bonus: Meditation and Mindfulness

Techniques: Developing Inner Calm and Resilience

Finding times of peace within the chaos of life can serve as a haven for the soul. We can develop inner calm, resilience, and presence via mindfulness and meditation techniques, which enable us to deal with the challenges of everyday life with grace and clarity. We'll examine the transforming potential of mindfulness and meditation in this investigation, as well as the significant ways in which these practices might improve our lives.

The Presence Art:

Earthing Breaths: Start by inhaling deeply a few times and letting the breath ground you in the here and now. Bring your entire awareness into the present now and pay attention to the feeling of air coming into and going out of your body. Feel yourself getting more focused and grounded with each breath, and as you exhale, feel tension and stress go.

Meditation using Body Scan: Gently scan your body from head to toe, noting any places of tension, discomfort, or ease. This is a journey of self-discovery. Gently become aware of the sensations you have with each breath, letting yourself inhabit your body completely in this very instant. Through developing an awareness of your body's knowledge, you can foster a more profound sense of presence and connection.

Developing Kindness and Compassion:

Meditation on Love and Kindness: Take a seat comfortably and think of a friend, relative, or mentor that you hold in high regard. Say loving-kindness affirmations to this individual with each breath, like "May you be happy, may you be healthy, may you be safe, may you be at peace." Send out these kind thoughts and wishes for compassion and kindness to everyone, acknowledging our connection and common humanity.

Practice Self-Compassion: Give yourself the same love and care that you would give to a close friend who is in need. Be mindful of any unease, self-criticism, or feelings of inadequacy, and respond to them with compassion and gentle curiosity. Remind yourself that you are loved and accepted just the way you are and that imperfections are a natural part of being human. Give yourself some words of consolation and assurance.

Silence in the Face of Chaos:

Cognitive Motion: Take up mild movement exercises like qigong, tai chi, or yoga, and let your body move naturally and gracefully. Pay close attention to how your body feels as you bend, stretch, and let go of tension during each exercise. Observe how movement can help you develop an inner sense of serenity and vitality, as well as assist you connect with the present moment, as it can be a sort of meditation.

Mindfulness in Nature: Go on a thoughtful stroll in the outdoors, letting your senses fully take in the sights, sounds, and textures of the surrounding environment. Take in the sights and sounds of the trees—the rustle of leaves in the breeze, the song of the birds. Give yourself over to the flow of life as it unfolds moment by moment and let nature lead the way. You will find peace and comfort in Mother Earth's embrace.

Letting Go and Accepting Impermanence:

Thoughts Raining Meditation: Think of your thoughts as softly falling raindrops from the sky, each one moving through your consciousness free from attachment or judgment. Examine the rise and fall of ideas, emotions, and experiences as they pass in and out like clouds in the sky. Find freedom and serenity in the spaciousness of consciousness by contenting yourself to just be a spectator to the constantly shifting terrain of your mind.

Practice Gratitude: By thinking back on the gifts and blessings in your life, both large and small, you can cultivate an attitude of thankfulness. Every day, set aside some time to reflect on the people, events, and occasions that enrich and deepen your life. You can open your heart to the richness and beauty of the present moment by practicing thankfulness, which will help you change your attention from what is lacking to what is abundant.

In conclusion, despite life's obstacles and uncertainties, mindfulness and meditation techniques provide a doorway to inner serenity, presence, and resilience. We can develop a stronger feeling of connection to ourselves, others, and the world around us by adopting these practices with an open heart and an inquiring mind. We can also find strength and comfort in the sanctuary of the present moment.

About the author,

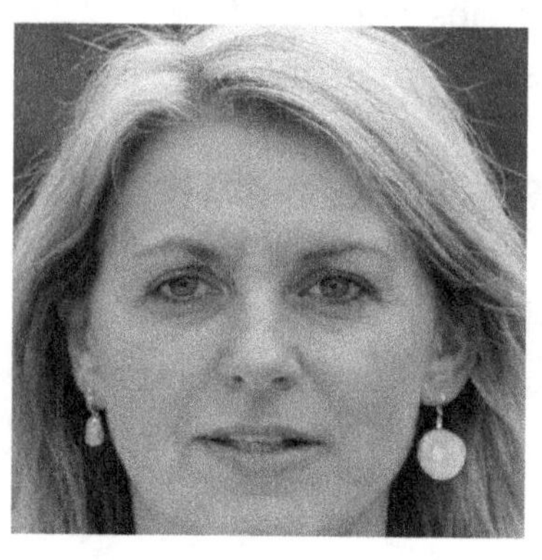

Teresa M. Broaddus is an ardent supporter of women's empowerment and health who has a profound awareness of the life-changing experience that is menopause. Teresa offers to her job a special fusion of understanding, skill, and compassion, drawing on both her professional and personal experiences.

Teresa, who has a background in wellness and healthcare, has made it her mission to help women navigate the opportunities and problems of menopause. As a licensed menopause educator and health coach, she has assisted many women in adjusting gracefully, resolutely, and vibrantly to this major life shift.

Teresa wants to enable women to see menopause as a period of personal development, change, and awakening. With her book "The Manifesto of Menopause," Teresa offers a thorough manual for handling the mental, emotional, and physical shifts that come with going through menopause with poise and confidence.

Teresa provides helpful guidance, empowering insights, and transformational practices to support women in thriving throughout this pivotal period, with an emphasis on holistic wellbeing and self-care. Teresa helps women to recover their health, vitality, and sense of purpose via her holistic approach to menopause, which includes mindfulness and meditation practices, nutrition advice, and self-care strategies.

Teresa wants to encourage women to perceive menopause as a chance for personal development, self-empowerment, and rejuvenation through her work. She leads women on a path of self-discovery and development with warmth, genuineness, and skill, assisting them in overcoming the obstacles of menopause with poise, fortitude, and hope.

Teresa M. Broaddus provides insight, direction, and empathy at every stage of the menopause, acting as a ray of hope and support for women navigating its difficulties. Her goal is to enable women to seize this pivotal period of life with resilience, joy, and confidence in order to maximize their potential for future growth, fulfillment, and well-being.

Table of content

Introduction

Embracing Change: A Journey of Acceptance

Change is an inevitable and constant force that shapes the very essence of our lives. It weaves through the tapestry of our existence, presenting itself in various forms, beckoning us to adapt, evolve, and grow. In the realm of personal transformation, few experiences carry as profound an impact as the intricate dance with change that menopause unfolds. This book, "The Manifesto of Menopause," is an invitation to explore the multifaceted landscape of this transformative journey, with a primary focus on accepting and embracing the changes that accompany this significant life stage.

The Nature of Change

Change, often synonymous with uncertainty, can evoke a spectrum of emotions. Menopause, as a natural biological process, heralds the cessation of menstrual cycles, symbolizing the end of one phase and the commencement of another. The emotional and physical shifts that accompany this transition can be both challenging and enlightening. It is crucial, however, to recognize that change is not synonymous with loss; rather, it is an opportunity for renewal, growth, and the unfolding of a new chapter.

In our modern society, menopause has been shrouded in myths and misconceptions, perpetuating a narrative that often casts it in a negative light. This introduction serves as a clarion call to reframe our understanding of menopause and to approach it with an open heart and a willingness to accept the changes it brings. As we embark on this exploration, let us delve into the intricacies of acceptance and the transformative power it holds.

The Power of Acceptance

Acceptance is not passive resignation but an active acknowledgment of reality—a conscious choice to engage with the present moment authentically. In the context of menopause, accepting the changes involves recognizing and embracing the fluctuations in hormonal balance, the physical alterations, and the evolving emotional landscape. This acceptance is not about erasing challenges but about building resilience and finding strength within the nuances of change.

This book unfolds a narrative that transcends mere acknowledgment, guiding you towards a profound acceptance of the menopausal journey. It is an affirmation that the power to shape your experience lies within your hands—a power that can be harnessed through understanding, knowledge, and intentional choices. By fostering an environment of acceptance, we pave the way for a transformative journey that transcends the limitations imposed by societal expectations and personal fears.

Navigating the Chapters

Each chapter within "The Manifesto of Menopause" is meticulously crafted to be a compass on this journey of acceptance. From the scientific underpinnings of menopause to the practical strategies for managing symptoms, from nutrition and fitness to mindfulness and holistic healing practices, every facet of the menopausal experience is explored. The chapters are designed to provide not only information but actionable steps, enabling you to navigate the changes with resilience, grace, and a sense of empowerment.

As you immerse yourself in the chapters that follow, consider this book as your companion—a guide that illuminates the path of acceptance. May it empower you to embrace the changes that menopause brings, recognizing them not as a diminishment but as a gateway to a richer, more fulfilling phase of life. Together, let us embark on this transformative journey of acceptance, forging a manifesto that celebrates the strength, wisdom, and beauty inherent in every woman's menopausal experience.

Recognize that menopause is a transforming experience.

Acknowledging Menopause as a Life-Changing Event.
Menopause is not only a biological phenomenon; rather, it is a deep and life-changing process that involves changes in one's physical, emotional, and spiritual development. When a woman's menstruation stops and a new chapter begins, it is a significant turning point in her life. This chapter explores the importance of understanding menopause as a period of transformation that goes beyond simple changes in hormone levels.

The Complex Character of Transformation

The menopause signals the end of the reproductive years and the beginning of a metamorphosis similar to the elegant change from a caterpillar to a butterfly. It's a natural, if sometimes difficult, evolution that asks women to release the reins of social expectations and accept the changing aspects of who they are. To acknowledge menopause as a transformational experience, it is necessary to examine its complex character and acknowledge not just the physical changes but also the accompanying emotional and psychological ones.

Handling Physical Shifts

Menopause's bodily changes serve as concrete reminders of the body's evolutionary history. Hormonal imbalances may cause symptoms including sleep problems, skin elasticity changes, and hot flashes. Recognizing these changes as signs of metamorphosis, as opposed to seeing them as minor inconveniences, may enable women to adjust and take better care of their bodies. The foundation of accepting the natural bodily transformation that comes with menopause is this realization.

Emotive Connection

Menopause is a journey, both physically and emotionally. Hormone fluctuations may affect mood, resulting in anything from intense feelings to periods of reflection. Acknowledging the complexities of one's emotions, accepting vulnerability, and cultivating a loving connection with oneself are all necessary to recognize the emotional resonance of menopause. Women may fully use the transforming potential of their menopausal experience by developing an emotional awareness.

Knowledge Revealed

Women who successfully traverse menopause start to accumulate a priceless store of knowledge. Menopause is a transforming event that reveals a depth of resilience, self-awareness, and understanding. It's an occasion to honor the abundance of life's experiences amassed over the years and to acknowledge the resilience that comes from enduring adversity. This acceptance of newly acquired knowledge is essential to changing menopause from a time of felt loss to one of great benefit.

An Introspective Journey

When menopause is seen as a life-changing event, it becomes a quest for personal growth. It's a chance to reevaluate priorities, discover interests, and reframe one's mission. The phases of menopause are not the conclusion of a tale; rather, they are the start of a new one, one that is molded by fortitude, sincerity, and a profound sense of self. Understanding menopause as a journey of transformation encourages women to take an active role in writing their own stories and to accept the layers of their identity that are changing.

Final Thought: The Transformation's Empowerment

In summary, menopause is a journey rather than a destination, one that calls on women to acknowledge and welcome the changes, both internal and external. It's an era of knowledge, self-awareness, and empowerment. Women may handle this life-changing period with grace, resilience, and a deep awareness of their power provided they accept the complex nature of menopause. I hope that this realization will serve as the impetus for a journey that honors the beauty that each woman's menopausal transformation.

Recognize the attitudes and stigmas that society has around menopause.

Exposing Stigmas and Attitudes in Society
Regarding Menopause
Menopause is a normal and unavoidable stage of a woman's life that is both a social and biological event. Menopause-related attitudes and stigmas have a big influence on how women see and handle this life-changing experience. This investigation explores the complex web of cultural viewpoints, exposing the misconceptions, prejudices, and stigmas that often cast a mist around menopause.

Mythologies and Inaccuracies

Myths and misunderstandings around menopause have long been spread by society, which has helped to create a negative cultural narrative about this time of life. Unfounded dread and anxiety may be instilled by myths such as the idea that a woman's beauty or usefulness ends with menopause. In order to remove the social hurdles preventing women from accepting menopause as a normal and empowered transition, it is imperative that these misconceptions be acknowledged.

The Mysteries Associated with Menopause

The general hush around menopause is one of the prevalent cultural views concerning it. In contrast to other life phases, menopause is sometimes shrouded in mystery, spoken about in whispers, or not talked about at all. This quiet might leave a gap where false information grows and make women feel alone in their experiences. Acknowledging this social stillness is the first move in encouraging candid conversation and eliminating the stigma around menopause.

Menopause and Ageism

The stigma attached to aging as a result of society's obsession with youth has contributed to ageism, a condition that has a direct bearing on how menopause is seen. Menopausal women may be marginalized by society's fixation on youth, which feeds the myth that becoming older makes one less valuable. A society that honors women at all stages of life, including menopause, must acknowledge and combat ageist beliefs.

Difficulties at Work

For women going through menopause, the workplace—a microcosm of cultural attitudes—often poses particular obstacles. Menopause-related attitudes that see it as a disability rather than a normal part of life might lead to prejudice at work and a lack of support. Advocating for workplace rules that recognize and accommodate the requirements of menopausal women requires an understanding of these problems.

Eliminating Stigmas with Teaching

Education turns as a potent weapon in the fight against menopausal stigmas. Through cultivating a culture of comprehension and consciousness, we may confront the assumed assumptions that sustain unfavorable perspectives. Realizing how important it is for everyone to know about menopause promotes a change in perspective toward a culture that values the fortitude and knowledge that women acquire from this life-changing event.

Encouraging Transformation

Acknowledging the stigmas and cultural views surrounding menopause is a call to action for empowerment and change rather than a means of maintaining victimization. It challenges these beliefs, calls for inclusion, and encourages women to take an active role in changing the narrative of culture. Women may take the lead in breaking down the social boundaries that have been built around the menopause as a normal and empowered stage in life.

Closing Remarks: A Request for Cultural Change

In summary, understanding social perceptions and stigmas related to menopause is crucial to promoting a cultural change. It demands candid discussion, instruction, and a team effort to rewrite the history of menopause. Our views of menopause should change along with society, moving from one of a stigmatized life period to one that is embraced for the resilience, power, and knowledge it bestows to women. I hope that this acknowledgment will serve as a spark for a more widespread social awareness, enabling women to accept menopause with dignity and genuineness.

Establish the tone for taking back authority over this phase of life.

Exposing Stigmas and Attitudes in Society Regarding Menopause

Menopause is a normal and unavoidable stage of a woman's life that is both a social and biological event. Menopause-related attitudes and stigmas have a big influence on how women see and handle this life-changing experience. This investigation explores the complex web of cultural viewpoints, exposing the misconceptions, prejudices, and stigmas that often cast a mist around menopause.

Mythologies and Inaccuracies

Myths and misunderstandings around menopause have long been spread by society, which has helped to create a negative cultural narrative about this time of life. Unfounded dread and anxiety may be instilled by myths such as the idea that a woman's beauty or usefulness ends with menopause. To remove the social hurdles preventing women from accepting menopause as a normal and empowered transition, these misconceptions must be acknowledged.

The Mysteries Associated with Menopause

The general hush around menopause is one of the prevalent cultural views concerning it. In contrast to other life phases, menopause is sometimes shrouded in mystery, spoken about in whispers, or not talked about at all. This quiet might leave a gap where false information grows and makes women feel alone in their experiences. Acknowledging this social stillness is the first move in encouraging candid conversation and eliminating the stigma around menopause.

Menopause and Ageism

The stigma attached to aging as a result of society's obsession with youth has contributed to ageism, a condition that has a direct bearing on how menopause is seen. Menopausal women may be marginalized by society's fixation on youth, which feeds the myth that becoming older makes one less valuable. A society that honors women at all stages of life, including menopause, must acknowledge and combat ageist beliefs.

Difficulties at Work

For women going through menopause, the workplace—a microcosm of cultural attitudes—often poses particular obstacles. Menopause-related attitudes that see it as a disability rather than a normal part of life might lead to prejudice at work and a lack of support. Advocating for workplace rules that recognize and accommodate the requirements of menopausal women requires an understanding of these problems.

Eliminating Stigmas with Teaching

Education turns as a potent weapon in the fight against menopausal stigmas. Through cultivating a culture of comprehension and consciousness, we may confront the assumed assumptions that sustain unfavorable perspectives. Realizing how important it is for everyone to know about menopause promotes a change in perspective toward a culture that values the fortitude and knowledge that women acquire from this life-changing event.

Encouraging Transformation

Acknowledging the stigmas and cultural views surrounding menopause is a call to action for empowerment and change rather than a means of maintaining victimization. It challenges these beliefs, calls for inclusion, and encourages women to take an active role in changing the narrative of culture. Women may take the lead in breaking down the social boundaries that have been built around menopause as a normal and empowered stage in life.

Closing Remarks: A Request for Cultural Change

In summary, understanding social perceptions and stigmas related to menopause is crucial to promoting cultural change. It demands candid discussion, instruction, and a team effort to rewrite the history of menopause. Our views of menopause should change along with society, moving from one of a stigmatized life period to one that is embraced for the resilience, power, and knowledge it bestows to women. I hope that this acknowledgment will serve as a spark for more widespread social awareness, enabling women to accept menopause with dignity and genuineness.

Chapter 1

Menopause's Scientific Basis

Changes in Hormones

The Scientific Basis of Menopause: Interpreting Hormone Changes

Menopause is a normal and unavoidable stage of a woman's life that is supported by a complex web of hormonal changes that affect both the body and the mind. This investigation explores the physiological underpinnings of menopause, revealing the subtleties of the hormonal shifts that characterize this life-changing experience.

The Hormonal Symphony of Menopause

The complex dance between progesterone, estrogen, and follicle-stimulating hormone (FSH) is the primary mechanism underlying the hormonal alterations that occur throughout menopause. These hormones are progressively produced less by the ovaries as a woman gets closer to menopause. A crucial component of the menstrual cycle, estrogen levels significantly drop, causing changes in monthly patterns and, in the end, the cessation of menstruation.

The Transition to Perimenopause

The perimenopausal transition, which usually begins in the late 30s or early 40s, is the first step on the path to menopause. Hormonal fluctuations intensify during this time, and women may encounter mood swings, hot flashes, and irregular menstruation cycles. As the ovaries become less receptive to hormonal feedback, FSH levels increase, signaling the onset of menopause.

Sub-Chapters:

1.Estrogen Decline:** - Examine how estrogen functions in the reproductive system of women.
   - Analyze how estrogen production decreases throughout the perimenopause.
   - Talk about how lower estrogen levels affect fertility and the menstrual cycle.

2. Changes in Progesterone:Recognize Progesterone's Function in the Menstrual Cycle.

Emphasize how progesterone levels fall during the perimenopause.
   - Talk about how progesterone fluctuations affect menopausal symptoms.

3. FSH: Follicle-stimulating hormone
   - Describe how FSH affects menstrual cycle regulation.
   Examine how perimenopausal rising FSH levels indicate ovarian decline.
   - Talk about the relationship between normal menopausal symptoms and FSH levels.

Analytical Impacts

Beyond the reproductive system, the menopausal hormone shifts have extensive physiological implications. The genitourinary system, cardiovascular health, and bones are some of the regions affected by the changed hormonal environment. Comprehending these physiological impacts offers a thorough perspective on menopause as an all-encompassing life transition.

Sub-Chapters:

1. Bone Health:Investigate the relationship between a decrease in estrogen and a loss of bone density.

- Talk about the heightened risk of osteoporosis both during and following menopause.
- Examine methods for preserving ideal bone health through interventions and lifestyle choices.

2. Cardiovascular Impact:Investigate the effect of estrogen in cardiovascular health.

Examine how postmenopausal women's hormonal fluctuations might raise their risk of cardiovascular disease.
- Talk about changing one's lifestyle to promote cardiovascular health throughout menopause.

3.Genitourinary Alterations: Analyze the effects of hormones on the genitourinary system.
- Talk about typical symptoms including dry vagina and changes in urination.

Examine methods for controlling genitourinary complaints to improve general well-being.

Effect on Emotional and Mental Health

Menopause-related hormonal changes might also have an impact on one's mental and emotional health. Anxiety, mood fluctuations, and cognitive alterations have all been related to variations in estrogen levels. Comprehending these associations illuminates the complex characteristics of the menopausal journey.

Sub-Chapters:

1. Anxiety and Mood Swings:
   Examine the connection between alterations in mood and variations in estrogen levels.
   - Talk about typical mood-related perimenopausal symptoms.
   - Emphasize techniques for handling anxiety and mood fluctuations.

2. Cognitive Changes:** - Examine how hormone fluctuations affect cognitive performance.
   Talk about cognitive issues including forgetfulness and trouble focusing.
   Investigate cognitive and lifestyle therapies to enhance menopausal cognitive health.

Final Thoughts: Getting Around the Hormone Landscape

In conclusion, the hormonal shifts that define this life-changing experience are deeply entwined with the scientific foundation of menopause. An understanding of the rise in FSH and the decrease in progesterone and estrogen lays the groundwork for understanding the effects on genitourinary, cardiovascular, physiological, and mental health. In addition to identifying changes, navigating the hormonal terrain of menopause involves arming women with the information they need to make decisions that will support their general well-being at this time of life transition. I hope that my investigation will help people better grasp the science underlying this normal and empowered stage of life by acting as a beacon of guidance through the hormonal complexities of menopause.

Examine how the body changes throughout menopause.

Managing the Shifts: Comprehending the Body's Metamorphosis During Menopause

Menopause, a turning point in a woman's life, brings with it a host of significant changes that go beyond changes in hormones. This investigation explores the complex web of changes that occur in the body during menopause, revealing the subtle physical aspects that influence this metamorphic experience.

The Menopause's Evolution

The body changes with the approach of menopause, denoting the end of the reproductive years. For women starting this journey, it is essential to comprehend these changes because they provide insights that promote acceptance, resiliency, and proactive self-care.

Changes in Menstruation and Stopping

Sub-Chapters:

1.Perimenopausal Transition: Examine the menstrual cycle irregularities associated with the perimenopausal phase.
  - Talk about the ways that variations in progesterone and estrogen affect menstruation patterns.
  - Offer an understanding of the emotional and psychological effects of switching from regular to irregular periods.

2.Menstruation Cessation: Recognize the biological causes of menstrual cessation.

- Talk about the mental and physical effects of menopausal women going through their final menstrual cycle.

Emphasize the importance of the postmenopausal stage for changes in reproduction.

Modifications to the Reproductive Organs

Reproductive organs undergo structural and functional changes throughout the menopausal transition. Comprehending these modifications facilitates the management of any obstacles and acceptance of the changing facets of reproductive health.

Sub-Chapters:

1. Ovarian Changes:nAnalyze how the loss of ovarian function affects the generation of hormones.

- Talk about the ovaries' function in menopause and their importance to the reproductive system as a whole.

Examine how ovarian alterations may affect hormone balance and fertility.

2. Changes in the Uterus and Vagina:

Examine how the tissues in the vagina and uterus alter as a woman goes through menopause.
 - Talk about typical symptoms including atrophy and dryness in the vagina.
Examine methods for supporting and maintaining vaginal health both during and after menopause.

Changes in Body Composition and Metabolism

Changes in body composition and metabolic processes frequently coincide with menopause. Making proactive lifestyle decisions that promote general health and well-being is made easier when one is aware of these changes.

Sub-Chapters:

1. Changes in Metabolism:
   Examine how menopausal hormone changes affect metabolism.
   - Talk about variations in energy expenditure and how they might affect controlling weight.
   - Emphasize how diet and exercise contribute to maintaining metabolic health.

2. Changes in Body Composition:
   Analyze variations in bone density, muscle mass, and fat distribution.

- Talk about the heightened risk of osteoporosis and methods for keeping bones healthy.

Examine how resistance training and exercise can help to mitigate changes in body composition.

Skin and Cardiovascular Changes

Skin vitality and cardiovascular health might be impacted by menopause. Women must be aware of these changes in order to proactively address their skincare and heart health concerns.

Sub-Chapters:

1. Changes in the Heart:
Examine how hormonal fluctuations affect the health of the cardiovascular system.
- Talk about the heightened risk of heart disease both during and beyond menopause.
Examine ways to improve your lifestyle to promote cardiovascular health.

2. Skin Aging: Analyze how estrogen contributes to the elasticity and moisture of the skin.
- Talk about typical menopausal skin changes, such as wrinkles and dryness.
Examine skin care procedures and treatments to enhance the health of your skin.

Concluding Remarks: Caring for the Body During Menopause

In summary, the body changes dramatically throughout menopause, including changes in the reproductive system, changes in the body's composition and metabolism, changes in the skin and cardiovascular system, and changes in menstruation. Comprehending these modifications enables women to traverse this path with expertise and elegance. Women who accept the subtle physical changes that come with menopause pave the way for proactive self-care, holistic well-being, and an appreciation of the strength that comes with each stage of life. I hope that my investigation will act as a roadmap, encouraging a more profound comprehension of the body's development and supporting women as they navigate the life-changing menopausal transition.

Recognize the effects on both mental and physical health

Nurturing the Whole Self: Understanding Menopause's Linked Effects on Mental and Physical Health

Menopause is a multi-faceted journey that deeply integrates mental and emotional health and goes beyond the boundaries of the physical world. This investigation unravels the complex tango between mind and body during this transitional time by exploring the interrelated impacts of menopause on mental and physical health.

Menopause's Mental Terrain

Sub-Chapters:

1. Emotional Flux and Mood Swings:
   - Investigate the impact of hormone variations on menopausal mood swings.
   - Talk about the emotional terrain characterized by times of resiliency and vulnerability.
   Examine techniques for controlling mood fluctuations and promoting mental health.

2. Cognitive and Anxiety Shifts:
   Examine the relationship between altered hormone levels and heightened anxiety susceptibility.

Examine cognitive alterations, such as forgetfulness and trouble focusing.
- Talk about cognitive techniques and lifestyle treatments that promote mental clarity and emotional stability.

Moving Through the Real Terrain

Sub-Chapters:

1. Sleep disturbances and hot flashes:
Examine how changes in hormones can cause physical symptoms like hot flashes.
- Talk about how sleep disruptions affect one's general physical health.
Emphasize dietary changes and good sleeping habits as ways to lessen these impacts.

2. Muscle Mass and Bone Health:
- Look into the connection between a decrease in estrogen and a decrease in bone density.
- Talk about how important it is to preserve bone health through activity and diet.
Examine the relationship between variations in muscle mass and strength and hormonal changes.

The Point Where Mental and Physical Health Intersect

Menopause is a point of intersection between physical and mental health, which interact in a complex and dynamic dance. It is crucial for women to comprehend this intersection in order to navigate the complex terrain of menopause.

Sub-Chapters:

1. Interplay between Stress and Hormones:**
   Examine how stress and hormone balance are related to one another.
   - Talk about the benefits of stress management for physical and mental health.
   Examine mindfulness techniques as strategies for promoting equilibrium in the face of stress.

2. Impact on Esteem and Self-Image:
   Analyze how society affects a woman's perception of herself during menopause.
   - Talk about the possible impacts on body image and self-esteem.
   - Emphasize methods for developing a positive view of oneself and accepting one's changing identity.

The Lifestyle as a Foundation for Health

Understanding how menopause affects one's physical and emotional health calls for a comprehensive approach to well-being. During this path of transformation, lifestyle decisions become crucial to supporting resilience and nourishing the full self.

 Sub-Chapters:

1. Nutrition and Hormonal Support:** - Examine how diet affects the balance of hormones throughout menopause.
   - Talk about particular nutrients that are necessary for both physical and mental health.
   - Emphasize eating habits that support general health at this period of life.

2. Using Your Body as a Catalyst:
   - Analyze the advantages of consistent exercise for hormonal balance and mental wellness.
   - Talk about specialized workout plans for ladies going through menopause.
   Examine how exercising might lessen menopausal symptoms on the physical and emotional levels.

Concluding Remarks: Adopting A Holistic Perspective

In conclusion, there is a call to embrace holistic well-being given the interrelated impacts of menopause on both physical and mental health. Understanding the dynamic interactions between mood and hormone swings, physical symptoms, and the impact of lifestyle choices is necessary for this journey. Many women choose to follow a path that emphasizes self-compassion, making educated decisions, and celebrating the robust full self that emerges through the menopausal landscape as they navigate this transitional era. I hope that our investigation will act as a guide and help people have a better grasp of the complex dance that menopause involves between physical and mental health.

Acknowledge that every woman's experience is unique.

Honoring Individuality: Recognizing the Diverse Fabric of Each Woman's Menopausal Journey

Each woman's menopause is a dramatic and transforming phase that creates a tapestry as unique as the lady going through it. This investigation explores the significance of recognizing and appreciating the uniqueness of each woman's menopausal experience in order to promote a supportive, empathetic, and empowered culture.

The Menopause's Complex Nature

Menopause is a complicated and multidimensional experience that includes emotional, psychological, and social aspects in addition to biological changes. Understanding that every woman embarks on this path with her unique history, viewpoints, and goals is essential to valuing the richness and diversity of the menopausal experience.

Genetics and Health History's Impact

Sub-Chapters:

1. **Genetic Variability:** - Examine how heredity influences the menopausal transition.
   - Talk about the ways that inherited patterns can affect the onset and signs of menopause.
   Stress how crucial it is to comprehend one's genetic heritage in order to foresee certain features of the menopausal experience.

2. Health History and Current Conditions:
   Analyze the potential effects of pre-existing medical issues on the menopausal experience.

- Talk about the impact of things like prescription drugs, lifestyle decisions, and chronic conditions.
- Stress the importance of individualized treatment plans based on each patient's unique medical background.

The Emotional Terrain: Viewpoints and Coping Strategies

Sub-Chapters:

1. Social and Cultural Factors:
   Examine how societal and cultural views affect people's perceptions of menopause.
   - Talk about how stigma, expectations, and cultural standards affect women's experiences.
   Stress the importance of having frank conversations in order to dispel myths and advance different points of view.

2. Resilience and Coping Mechanisms:
   Examine the variety of coping strategies used by women going through menopause.
   - Talk about the ways that coping mechanisms, support networks, and personal resilience affect the emotional journey.
   Emphasize the value of identifying and discussing a range of coping strategies.

Personal Preferences & Lifestyle

Sub-Chapters:

1. Variety of Lifestyle Options:
   Examine the differences in women's lifestyle choices with regard to nutrition, exercise, and stress reduction.
   - Talk about how these decisions affect managing symptoms and general well-being.
   Stress the need for customized lifestyle strategies that suit individual tastes.

2. Perceptions of Hormonal Treatments:
   - Look into how women feel about and would like to use hormone therapy.
   - Talk about the various viewpoints on alternative therapies and hormone replacement therapy (HRT).
   - Promote well-informed decision-making that is consistent with personal views and comfort zones.

Effect on Support Networks and Relationships

Sub-Chapters:

1. Varied Relationship Dynamics:

Examine the ways in which menopause affects friendships, family dynamics, and partnerships.
   - Talk about the various ways that support networks and significant others either exacerbate or lessen menopausal symptoms.
   Stress the value of open communication and understanding in interpersonal relationships.

2. Personal Networks' Role:
   Examine how social networks affect how one experiences menopause.
   - Talk about the benefits of mentorship, online groups, and friendships for support and knowledge sharing.
   Stress the power that comes from having a varied and welcoming community.

Final Thoughts: Accepting Variety in the Menopausal Mosaic

In conclusion, recognizing the individuality of each woman's menopausal experience is a call to enjoy the diversity found in the mosaic of menopause. Many women find strength in their unique stories as they travel through this life-changing experience and realize that there is no one-size-fits-all approach to menopause. Menopausal experiences are a rich and diverse tapestry that should be honored, respected, and celebrated. I hope that this investigation will serve as a reminder of the beauty and power that come from accepting each woman's menopausal experience as unique.

Myths About Menopause Busted

Lifting the Veil: Busting Myths Regarding Menopause

Menopause is a normal and unavoidable stage of a woman's life, but there are many myths and misconceptions around it that make it difficult to understand this life-changing experience. In order to promote a more truthful and powerful narrative that is in line with the realities of this important life stage, this investigation seeks to expose and debunk prevalent myths surrounding menopause.

Myth 1: Aging and Decline are Indicated by Menopause

Menopause is often associated with aging and decline, which feeds into a negative stereotype. Menopause is actually a normal biological process rather than a sign of lost significance or usefulness.

By dispelling this myth, women are encouraged to see menopause as a change that heralds a new and potentially rewarding stage of life that is characterized by resilience, knowledge, and personal development.

Myth 2: Every Woman Goes Through Menopause Differently

Sub-Chapters:

1. Varieties of Experiences:- Examine the wide range of menopausal experiences that women have.
   - Talk about the menopause's duration, age of onset, and symptom differences.
   Stress how important it is to acknowledge and value the uniqueness of every woman's path.

2. Personalized Methods:
   Emphasize the necessity of individualized methods for the treatment of menopausal symptoms.
   - Talk about how individual experiences are influenced by lifestyle decisions, attitudes, and medical history.
   - Motivate medical professionals to deliver tailored advice and assistance.

Myth 3: Hot Flashes Are the Only Symptom of Menopause

Even if hot flashes are a typical symptom, menopause is too complicated to be reduced to just one element. Numerous physical, emotional, and psychological changes are associated with menopause. By dispelling this myth, we may better comprehend menopause and promote a more comprehensive strategy for navigating the intricacies of this time of life.

Myth 4: There is an Irreversible Physical and Mental Decline During Menopause

Sub-Chapters:

1. Adopting Positive Aging:Disprove the idea that menopause equates to irreversible aging.
   - Talk about how having a good outlook on life might affect how aging is seen.
   - Draw attention to the experiences of women who have accepted menopause as a period of rebirth and empowerment.

2. Importance of Maintaining Health:
Stress the need to take preventative health steps to lessen age-related changes.

- Talk about how diet, exercise, and lifestyle choices all contribute to general well-being.

- Motivate women to place a high priority on maintaining their health both throughout and after menopause.

Myth 5: The Only Treatment for Menopausal Symptoms Is Hormonal Therapy

The misconception that hormonal therapies are the only choice for treating symptoms is oversimplified, even if they can be useful in managing symptoms. In order to dispel this notion, a variety of strategies must be investigated, such as non-hormonal drugs, alternative therapies, and lifestyle changes, to give women a complete toolset for handling their particular menopausal experiences.

Myth 6: Talking about menopause is taboo

Sub-Chapters:

1. Encouraging Open Discussion:Analyze the social and cultural elements that contribute to the stigma associated with menopause.

- Talk about how important it is to promote frank and open discussions on menopause.

- Encourage women to talk about their experiences in order to normalize conversations about this normal stage of life and to remove stigma.

2. Educational Initiatives Promote menopausal education in businesses, educational institutions, and healthcare settings.
   - Talk about how raising awareness can help dispel myths and create a welcoming atmosphere.
   Stress how important it is for the media to appropriately and favorably represent menopause.

Final Thought: Using Truth to Empower Women

In summary, busting stereotypes around menopause is essential to educating women, giving them correct information, and creating a friendly atmosphere. We can help bring about a societal shift that celebrates menopause as a normal and transformative time by fighting misconceptions, supporting diversity, and encouraging candid conversation. I hope that this investigation can act as a spark to blow away the myths and empower women to face menopause with resilience, confidence, and a better knowledge of their own special experiences.

Dispel misunderstandings that are often held about menopause.

Revealing Objectivity: Eliminating Frequently Held Myths Regarding Menopause

Menopause is a normal stage of a woman's life that is sometimes clouded in misconceptions that feed into stereotypes and cause unwarranted fear. By shedding light on common misunderstandings about menopause, this investigation aims to promote a more knowledgeable and encouraging view of this life-changing experience.

Misconception 1: Menopause is a One-Time Event

Sub-Chapters:

1. Understanding the Transition: - Make it clear that menopause is a process of transition rather than a single event.
   - Talk about the phases, such as the menopause, postmenopause, and perimenopause.
   - Emphasize that years before menopause, during the perimenopause, menopausal symptoms can start.

2. Variability in Onset: - Examine the variations in women's menopausal onset ages.
   - Talk about the lifestyle, health history, and genetics that affect the time.
   - Stress that there is no set age for menopause; rather, it is a personal journey for each woman.

 Misconception 2: Reproductive Health Is the Only Affected Aspect of Menopause

Menopause is characterized by the end of menstrual cycles, but its effects go well beyond reproductive health. Clearing up this misconception requires acknowledging that menopause is a comprehensive process that includes physical, emotional, and psychological elements.

 Misconception 3: All Menopausal Symptoms Are Severe

Sub-Chapters:

1. Difference in Symptoms
   - Make clear that menopausal symptoms differ greatly from woman to woman.
   - Talk about typical symptoms including mood swings, heat flashes, and insomnia.

Emphasize that although some women may have few or no symptoms, others may have more severe ones.

2. Standard of Symptoms: - Dispel the myth that menopausal symptoms last forever.
Talk about the transient nature of many symptoms and how long they last.
- Stress that coping mechanisms and support-seeking can greatly reduce the intensity of symptoms.

Misconception 4: Sexual Well-Being Is Ended with Menopause

Sub-Chapters:

1. Impact on Libido:- Dispel the myth that a decrease in libido is an inevitable consequence of menopause.
- Talk about the psychological and biological variables that affect changes in sexual desire.
- Stress that, with the right communication and flexibility, it is possible to preserve sexual well-being during menopause.

2. Tackling intimate Issues: - Make it clear that menopause may cause intimate issues, but that communication is essential.
   - Talk about typical problems, such as vaginal dryness and discomfort, and possible fixes.
   - To address intimacy difficulties, promote candid communication with partners and healthcare professionals.

 Misunderstanding 5: The Only Remedy Is Hormonal Therapy

Although hormone therapies have their place, the idea that they are the only option must be refuted. By making the spectrum of possibilities more clear, women are better equipped to make decisions based on their personal preferences and needs.

Misconception 6: Gaining Weight Is Inevitable During Menopause

Sub-Chapters:

1. Metabolic Changes: - Dispel the myth that weight gain is an inevitable consequence of menopause.
   - Talk about the effects of hormones on body composition and metabolism.

Stress the importance of lifestyle decisions, such as nutrition and exercise, in controlling weight throughout menopause.

2. Empowering Body Positivity:- Talk about the preconceptions and social pressures associated with menopause-related body image.
   - Talk about how important it is to embrace self-acceptance and body positivity.
   - Encourage women to put more emphasis on their general health and well-being than on meeting irrational expectations.

Concluding Remarks: Encouraging Women via Knowledge

In summary, clearing up misconceptions regarding menopause is essential to enabling women to take charge of this life-changing process and do so with confidence and understanding. We add to a more knowledgeable and encouraging narrative about menopause by elucidating the stages, variety of symptoms, impact on sexual well-being, and accessible management options. I hope that my investigation will act as a guide, promoting a deeper comprehension and tearing down the falsehoods that have masked the actual nature of this healthy and empowering stage of life.

Contest cultural narratives

Tackling Cultural Narratives: An Appeal to Dispel Myths and Promote Understanding

Cultural narratives about many facets of life frequently influence our viewpoints and actions, but they can also reinforce preconceptions and misconceptions. This investigation explores the significance of challenging cultural narratives and promoting a critical analysis of deeply held convictions to promote a more inclusive, enlightened, and compassionate understanding.

Breaking Down Cultural Myths

Sub-Chapters:

1. The Power of Cultural Narratives:
Recognize how cultural narratives shape society perceptions.
   - Talk about the ways that cultural narratives influence the development of expectations, values, and standards.

Stress how important it is to carefully examine these stories to find hidden prejudices and disprove long-held notions.

2. Identifying preconceptions: Examine prevalent preconceptions that are woven into cultural stories.
   - Talk about how these prejudices harm vulnerable populations and uphold social injustices.
   Emphasize how awareness and critical thinking are essential for spotting and dispelling damaging stereotypes.

Challenging Gender Preconceptions

Cultural narratives frequently uphold strict gender rules that restrict personal expression and bolster inequity. It is crucial to challenge these myths to promote gender equality and destroy damaging preconceptions.

Sub-Chapters:

1. Reimagining norms: - Question the societal narratives that uphold established gender norms.
   - Talk about how important it is to accept different gender identification manifestations.
   Emphasize stories that defy restrictive stereotypes and advance empowerment and inclusivity.

2. Intersectionality: - Recognize that identities, such as those about race, gender, and sexual orientation, are intersecting.

- Challenge narratives that minimize or oversimplify the experiences of people whose identities cross.

- Promote narratives that honor the diversity and complexity of many life experiences.

Challenging Cultural Plunder

Sub-Chapters:

1. Understanding Appropriation:- Explain what cultural appropriation is and how it affects underprivileged groups.

Talk about situations where cultural customs are commercialized without regard for cultural sensitivity or propriety.

- Stress how important it is to respect and acknowledge the cultural roots of customs and behaviors.

2. Encouraging Cultural Exchange:- Distinguish between authentic cultural exchange and appropriation.

- Promote stories that honor the traditions'
historical context while showcasing cultural variety.
   Emphasize the benefits of genuine cross-cultural
understanding for promoting world peace.

Challenging Ageism

Cultural narratives frequently reinforce age-related
biases and preconceptions. To combat ageism, one
must question these myths and acknowledge the
diversity and importance of life experiences at all
phases.

Sub-Chapters:

1. Redefining Aging:- Disprove myths that
characterize aging as a downward spiral.
   Emphasize the wisdom and wealth that aging
brings.
   - Promote narratives that reinterpret aging as a
progression of development and contribution.

2. Intergenerational Connections: Examine stories
that encourage cooperation and understanding
between generations.
   - Talk about the advantages of encouraging
relationships between various age groups.

- Highlight the knowledge and experiences that cross-generational connections can impart.

Challenging Social Myths Regarding Mental Health

Sub-Chapters:

1. Breaking the Silence: Disprove cultural myths that stigmatize mental illness.
   - Talk about how having candid discussions helps to lessen stigma.
   - Promote stories that empathetically and sympathetically portray mental health issues.

2. Encouraging Mental Wellness: - Examine cultural narratives that encourage self-care and mental wellness.
   - Talk about how storytelling contributes to the development of a positive cultural environment.
   Stress the importance of truthful and sympathetic representations of experiences with mental health.

Final Thoughts: Crafting Inclusive Storylines

In summary, challenging cultural narratives is a crucial first step in creating a society that is more compassionate, understanding, and inclusive. Our efforts to dispel the stigma around mental health, confront ageism, confront stereotypes, and address appropriation help to build cultural narratives that represent the variety and depth of human experience. I hope that my investigation will function as a spark for people to actively challenge damaging narratives and take part in weaving together a cultural fabric that values and celebrates the diversity of voices and stories.

Promote a knowledgeable and independent strategy

Strengthening Self-reliance: Encouraging Informed and Self-Acting Approaches

Promoting an informed and autonomous approach becomes essential for decision-making, critical thinking, and personal development in an information-rich society. This investigation explores the need to promote a methodology that unites the acquisition of knowledge with the independence to create own ideas, make thoughtful decisions, and negotiate life's intricacies.

The Age of Excessive Information

Sub-Chapters:

Firstly, Navigating Information Highways:-
Recognize how much information is available in the digital age.
   - Talk about the difficulties of identifying trustworthy sources in the deluge of available data.
   - Stress the importance of people learning how to evaluate information and think critically.

2. Sifting Through the Noise:- Examine methods for sifting through pertinent data and evaluating its reliability.
   - Talk about the consequences of false information and the significance of fact-checking.
   - Encourage people to choose their sources of information with an emphasis on diversity and dependability.

Fostering an Informed Mentality

Sub-Chapters:

1. Lifetime Learning Philosophy:- Promote a lifetime learning philosophy as the cornerstone of knowledge acquisition.

- Talk about the advantages of adaptability, curiosity, and a hunger for information for both professional and personal growth.

Emphasize the notion that learning comes from a variety of sources and experiences and goes beyond formal schooling.

2. Cross-Disciplinary Understanding: - Encourage people to learn about topics from other fields of study.

- Talk on the importance of cross-disciplinary understanding and the interconnectedness of information.

Stress that a comprehensive understanding of the world encourages original thought and diverse viewpoints.

Developing Critical and Analytical Thinking Capabilities

Sub-Chapters:

1. Analyzing Information: - Talk about how critical it is to have analytical abilities in order to analyze complicated data.

Investigate methods for dissecting information into digestible parts.

- Encourage people to critically assess the facts and pose questions about presumptions.

2. Capacity for Solving Problems:
  - Draw attention to the link between knowledge and practical problem-solving.
  - Talk about how developing solutions requires both analytical and creative thinking.
  Promote the application of knowledge to practical problems.

Promoting Independence and Autonomy

Sub-Chapters:

1. Informed Decision-Making: - Promote the idea that having information and being able to make informed decisions are related.
  - Talk about the empowerment that results from being able to comprehend and evaluate options.
  Stress how crucial it is to take into account a variety of viewpoints while making decisions.

2. Autonomy in Personal Growth: - Examine the ways in which autonomy promotes self-awareness and personal development.
  - Talk about how independence shapes a person's identity and morals.

- Motivate people to pursue information that is consistent with their own objectives and desires.

A Guide to Handling Ethical Issues

Sub-Chapters:

1. Ethical Information Consumption: - Talk about the moral obligations pertaining to acquiring knowledge.
   Examine how information intake affects society's viewpoints.
   - Encourage individuals to consider the ethical implications of their knowledge-seeking behaviors.

2. Contributing Positively to Discourse:
   - Highlight the role of informed individuals in fostering positive discourse.
   - Discuss strategies for engaging in discussions with respect, empathy, and openness.
   - Stress how knowledgeable people can help bring about constructive changes in society.

 Conclusion: Empowered by Knowledge, Driven by Independence

In conclusion, promoting a knowledgeable and independent strategy is pivotal for navigating the complexities of the modern world. Through the development of a lifelong learning mindset, the enhancement of critical thinking abilities, the promotion of autonomy, and the contemplation of ethical issues, people can enable themselves to make well-informed decisions, make constructive contributions to society, and continuously progress on their spiritual and intellectual paths. May this exploration serve as a guide, inspiring individuals to embrace the synergy between knowledge and independence, and to embark on a path of continuous growth, understanding, and self-discovery.

Chapter 2

Getting Around the Symptoms

It can be a complex road to manage menopause symptoms, involving self-care routines, lifestyle changes, and perhaps medication interventions. Maintaining general well-being becomes increasingly dependent on recognizing and treating the wide range of symptoms that women experience as they move through this transitional stage.

Hot flashes, which are characterized by intense heat waves that can cause discomfort and perspiration, are typical menopausal symptoms. Keeping cool surroundings, dressing in breathable materials, and engaging in relaxation exercises like deep breathing or meditation can all help to relieve symptoms. Hot flashes may also be controlled by eating a balanced diet high in fruits, vegetables, and whole grains and limiting caffeine and alcohol.

Menopause-related sleep disorders present additional difficulty. Better sleep quality can be achieved by establishing a regular sleep schedule, making your bedroom cozy, and avoiding stimulating activities just before bed. To encourage a more restful night's sleep, some ladies find comfort through relaxation exercises like moderate yoga or meditation.

During the menopause, mood swings and emotional disturbances are normal. Regular physical activity helps improve mood and general mental health, whether it be swimming, walking, or other low-impact activities. An avenue for emotional expression and coping mechanisms can also be found in the support of friends, family, or a mental health professional.

Menopause may bring on cognitive abnormalities, commonly known as "brain fog." Maintaining mental stimulation through puzzles, reading, or picking up new skills is crucial to improving cognitive function. A balanced diet and enough sleep are two more factors that support cognitive wellness.

Because menopause lowers estrogen levels, which increases the risk of osteoporosis, bone health is a worry. Bone health can be supported by including weight-bearing activities like strength training and walking, as well as consuming enough calcium and vitamin D. To monitor bone density and address any potential abnormalities, routine check-ups with healthcare specialists are needed.

Often, treating symptoms requires working with medical professionals. Under the supervision of their healthcare physician, some women may choose to undergo Hormone Replacement Therapy (HRT). HRT might not be appropriate for everyone, so it's important to consider the risks as well as the possible advantages.

In summary, managing menopausal symptoms requires a customized approach that considers both physical and mental health holistically. Women can move through this transformative time with strength and empowerment if they adopt a healthy lifestyle, seek assistance, and explore medical interventions when needed.

Physical Modifications

Menopause-related physical changes include adjustments to many parts of a woman's body. Maintaining general physical well-being requires identifying and treating these variations, which range from changes in weight distribution to changes in skin health and muscle tone.

One obvious physical alteration that occurs during menopause is a change in body composition, which is sometimes accompanied by weight increase, particularly in the abdominal area. This is caused in part by lifestyle choices, impaired metabolism, and hormonal swings. Regular physical activity can help control weight and improve general health. Examples of this type of exercise include cardiovascular and strength training. It is similarly necessary to choose a diet rich in nutrients and well-balanced to help the body adjust to these changes.

During menopause, skin modifications are also prevalent. Skin elasticity and moisture might be lost as a result of decreased collagen production. Women can think about using skincare regimens that incorporate sun protection and hydrating products to address this. Maintaining the health of your skin requires drinking enough water to hydrate your body from the inside out. A dermatologist consultation might offer specific recommendations for skincare products appropriate for menopausal skin.

A feeling of stiffness or soreness may be attributed to changes in the muscles and joints. Regularly stretching or doing yoga are good ways to preserve joint mobility and release tension in the muscles. Strength training helps maintain general physical function and preserve muscular mass. Furthermore, consuming anti-inflammatory foods like nuts and fish, which are high in omega-3 fatty acids, can help reduce joint pain.

The menopause affects bone health as well; a decrease in estrogen levels raises the risk of osteoporosis. Maintaining bone density requires weight-bearing activities like walking and resistance training. To maintain bone health, one must consume enough calcium and vitamin D through food or supplements. Frequent bone density evaluations with medical professionals can aid in tracking alterations and quickly addressing any issues.

Menopause also causes changes in hair, such as variations in thickness and texture. Maintaining the health of your hair requires eating a diet that is well-balanced and rich in essential vitamins and minerals, such as iron and biotin. Minimizing damage can be achieved by avoiding excessive heat styling and using gentle hair care products.

In conclusion, there are a variety of intricate physical changes that occur throughout menopause. A comprehensive strategy that includes consistent exercise, a healthy diet, skincare routines, and talks with medical experts can enable women to face these transitions with fortitude and self-assurance. An important part of the menopausal journey is coming to terms with and accepting one's changing physical self.

Take care of typical bodily complaints

Taking care of a variety of symptoms that differ from woman to woman is necessary while managing common physical issues during menopause. Knowing how to handle common issues like vaginal dryness and hot flashes is crucial to improving general health and quality of life.

Hot flashes, which are marked by erratic heat waves and perspiration, are a common menopausal symptom. Fans, layering clothing, and keeping a cool environment can all help manage them. Relaxation methods like mindfulness meditation and deep breathing help some women feel better. Limiting triggers like caffeine, alcohol, and spicy meals may also help reduce the frequency of hot flashes.

Hormonal changes during menopause often cause vaginal dryness and discomfort. During intimate moments, using lubricants with silicone or water bases can help. Regular stimulation or sexual activity can help preserve vaginal health by increasing blood flow to the region. Speaking with a healthcare professional might help you find specialized answers for ongoing problems, such as hormone therapy or other treatments.

Common problems include sleep disorders such as sleeplessness and night sweats. Better sleep quality can be achieved by establishing a regular sleep schedule, making your bedroom cozy, and avoiding stimulants like caffeine just before bed. Moreover, calming herbal teas or meditation are examples of relaxation methods that might help encourage sound sleep.

Menopause-related mood swings and irritability can be difficult. Regular exercise, like yoga or walking, releases endorphins, which have a favorable effect on mood. Making connections with loved ones, friends, or support groups can serve as a therapeutic outlet. For more persistent mental issues, therapy or counseling may be helpful in certain situations.

Menopause can cause pain in the muscles and joints. Regular exercise, which includes strength and cardiovascular training, can help reduce these discomforts. For further relief, try warm compresses, massages, and over-the-counter painkillers. It is best to speak with a healthcare professional if your pain is severe or chronic.

During menopause, weight gain is a major problem. Maintaining a healthy weight requires eating a balanced diet high in fruits, vegetables, and whole grains. Frequent exercise, including aerobic and strength training activities, can help preserve muscle mass and increase metabolism. Consulting with a dietitian or other medical professional might yield individualized weight-management plans.

Cognitive alterations and memory loss, commonly known as "brain fog," can happen. Learning new skills or solving puzzles are examples of mental workouts that might support cognitive function. In addition, stress reduction and getting enough sleep are essential for cognitive health. Speaking with a medical expert can help rule out underlying problems if worries continue.

In summary, managing common physical symptoms during menopause entails a mix of dietary changes, self-care routines, and, if required, medicinal measures. By being aware of and responding to these prevalent worries, women are better equipped to move through this stage with fortitude and a proactive attitude toward their general health and well-being.

Give useful advice for symptom management.

A comprehensive strategy that takes into account lifestyle modifications, self-care routines, and, when required, medical interventions is crucial to effectively manage menopausal symptoms. Here are some helpful tips for managing symptoms during this time of transformation:

1. Healthy Living Options:
   - Make the switch to a diet high in fruits, vegetables, whole grains, lean proteins, and well-balanced foods. This can promote general health, supply necessary nutrients, and aid with weight management.
   - Make sure you consume enough water throughout the day to stay hydrated. Drinking

enough water is essential for several body processes and can improve skin health.

- Take part in regular physical activity, which should include strength and cardio training. Exercise improves mood, encourages better sleep, and aids with weight management.

2. Temperature Regulation: - Wear layers to readily react to temperature variations during hot flashes. Make use of fans or leave windows open to keep the atmosphere cool. Recognize and stay away from hot flash causes, such as spicy meals, coffee, and alcohol.

3. Sleep Hygiene: - Create a regular sleep schedule by settling in and waking up at the same time every day.

- Keep the bedroom cold, quiet, and dark to create a good sleeping environment.

- Minimize screen time before bed because blue light from electronics might disrupt your sleep.

4. Social Welfare:

- Use stress-reduction strategies to control mood swings and irritation, such as deep breathing, mindfulness, or meditation.

- Make connections with loved ones, friends, or support groups to exchange stories and get moral support.

- If mood swings or emotional issues are persistent, think about getting treatment or counseling.

5. Intimate Health:- To relieve vaginal dryness during intimate times, use lubricants with silicone or water bases.

Make regular intercourse a priority to preserve the health of your vagina and the blood flow to that area.

See a doctor for individualized treatment plans, like as hormone therapy, if you have ongoing intimate health issues.

6. Cognitive Health: - Practice your cognitive function by doing puzzles, reading, or picking up new skills.

- Make sure you get enough sleep, as it is essential for maintaining good memory and cognitive function.

- Control stress by using relaxation methods to lessen the effects of "brain fog."

7. Medical Interventions: - Seek the counsel of medical specialists for tailored guidance and possible medical interventions.

Under the supervision of a healthcare professional, hormone replacement therapy (HRT) may be investigated after a risk-benefit analysis.

- Routine examinations and screenings can support the monitoring of general health, cardiovascular risk, and bone health.

Keep in mind that each person's menopausal experience is unique, so what works for one may not work for another. It's crucial to pay attention to your body, make self-care a priority, and seek advice from medical specialists for specific recommendations based on your particular requirements and worries.

Emphasize the value of practicing self-care and mental health ealth

Stressing the need for self-care is essential throughout the transitional stage of menopause, especially when it comes to mental health. Making self-care a priority grows increasingly important as women manage physical and hormonal changes and become more powerful in preserving their general well-being.

1. Comprehending Menopausal Mental Health:
   - Recognize how menopause-related hormonal changes affect one's emotional state and mood.
   Acknowledge the connection between physical and hormonal changes and mental health, highlighting the significance of a comprehensive approach to self-care.

2. The Significance of Self-Care for Mental Wellness:
   - Taking care of oneself is essential, particularly during menopause. It is not a luxury. Making time for oneself can have a big impact on mental clarity and emotional toughness.
   Making self-care a priority promotes optimism and lowers stress and anxiety, which are frequently linked to menopausal symptoms.

3. Mindfulness and Stress Reduction- Include mindfulness exercises in regular routines, including deep breathing exercises, meditation, or mindful walking. These techniques can aid in stress management, strengthen emotional control, and increase mental health in general.

4. Healthy Lifestyle Choices:- Adopt a diet rich in nutrients, such as omega-3 fatty acids, which are found in walnuts, flaxseeds, and seafood, that boost brain health.

Frequent exercise improves physical health and releases endorphins, which lift spirits and lessen depressive and anxious symptoms.

5. Quality Sleep for Mental Well-Being: - Make maintaining proper sleep hygiene a priority to have deep, revitalizing sleep.

- The correlation between insufficient sleep and mood swings, irritation, and cognitive difficulties highlights the need for getting enough sleep for mental well-being.

6. Connection and Support:- Encourage the development of relationships with loved ones, friends, or support groups to exchange stories and offer consolation.

- Having an open dialogue about menopausal experiences fosters a supportive community and works to dispel the stigma associated with mental health issues.

7. Professional Guidance:- If you're having trouble with any particular mental health issues, think about getting professional assistance, like therapy

or counseling. Skilled experts can help with negotiating the emotional difficulties of menopause, offer coping mechanisms, and create a safe environment for emotional expression.

8. Setting Limits and Setting Yourself First:
   - Set up sensible boundaries to control tension and avoid burnout.
   - Make self-care activities a priority without feeling guilty about it, realizing that mental health care improves one's general quality of life.

9. Mind-Body Connection: - Learn about mind-body techniques that combine physical exercise and mindfulness, such as yoga or tai chi, to promote a comprehensive strategy for both physical and mental well-being.

In conclusion, stressing the need for self-care is crucial for navigating this life-changing stage with resilience and grace, particularly when it comes to mental health during menopause. Women who prioritize self-care are better able to handle stress, have a positive outlook, and improve their emotional health—all of which will lead to a happier and healthier menopausal journey.

Managing Emotional Challenges Throughout Menopause:

1. Mood Swings and Irritability: - Hormonal changes associated with menopause frequently cause mood swings and irritability.
   - Mindfulness practices like deep breathing or meditation, as well as keeping lines of communication open with loved ones, are examples of coping mechanisms.

2. Stress and Anxiety: - Menopause-related bodily changes and uncertainties can lead to stress and anxiety.
   - Reduction of stress can be achieved by regular exercise and reaching out to friends or therapy for support.

3. Depression and Emotional Lows:- Feelings of melancholy or depression may be brought on by hormonal changes and the psychological effects of menopausal symptoms. It is imperative to seek professional assistance, such as therapy or

counseling, to address and manage these emotional lows.

4. Body image and self-esteem issues:
  - Self-esteem and body image may be affected by changes in body composition and how aging is perceived.
  - These issues can be resolved by embracing a good self-image, taking part in joyful activities, and asking for assistance.

5. Impact on partnerships: - Communication problems or estrangement might result from emotional troubles in partnerships.
  - Relationships can be strengthened during this time by being open and honest with partners and loved ones, expressing needs, and asking for understanding.

6. Loss and Grieving:Menopause can be linked to feelings of loss, such as the end of fertility and aging-related bodily changes. Emotional healing begins with acknowledging these losses and permitting oneself to grieve.

7. Cognitive alterations and irritation: Feelings of mental exhaustion and "brain fog" might result in cognitive alterations and irritation.

- Developing coping strategies, such as routine organization and patience exercises, can aid in the management of cognitive difficulties.

8. Fear of the Unknown:- Menopause is a major life shift, and worry and fear might arise from not knowing what is ahead.
    - Reassurance can be obtained through learning about menopause, consulting medical specialists, and making connections with other women who have experienced similar things.

Coping Techniques:

1. Open Communication: Talk to family, friends, or a support group about your feelings and experiences. It can be reassuring to know you are not alone in your challenges.

2. Seek specialist Support: To manage difficult emotions with the help of a qualified specialist, think about therapy or counseling.

3. Mindfulness and Relaxation Techniques: To reduce stress and improve emotional well-being, include mindfulness exercises in your daily routine, such as meditation or deep breathing techniques.

4. Physical Activity:- Studies have indicated that regular exercise improves mood and lessens depressive and anxious symptoms. Whether it's dancing, yoga, or strolling, find things you enjoy doing.

5. Grace for Oneself:- During this time of transition, treat yourself with kindness. Recognize your feelings and allow yourself the grace to work through them.

Recall that emotional difficulties are normal and acceptable throughout the menopause. Since every person's experience is different, it's important to figure out what coping strategies and support networks are most effective for you to promote mental health during this momentous life shift.

Describe coping techniquesPromote candid dialogue and asking for help.

Managing Strategies for Menopausal Difficulties:

Many physical and psychological changes coincide with menopause, and learning healthy coping mechanisms is essential to getting through this life-changing stage. These coping mechanisms can assist people in managing the difficulties associated with menopause:

1. Promote Self-Care: - Give self-care activities that make you happy and relaxed top priority. Some examples of these activities include reading, having a warm bath, or doing your favorite pastime.
   - Consistently evaluate and attend to individual requirements, stressing the significance of preserving mental and emotional health.

2. Telaxation and Mindfulness Methods:
   - Use mindfulness techniques to reduce stress and foster calmness, such as meditation or deep breathing exercises.
   - Engaging in mindful practices such as yoga or tai chi can improve the mind-body connection and promote general well-being.

3. Healthy Lifestyle Options: To support general health and energy levels, adopt a nutrient-rich, well-balanced diet.
   - Frequent physical activity can help control weight, elevate mood, and enhance sleep. This includes both aerobic and strength training.

4. Rstablish Supportive Routines Make sleep, exercise, and relaxation the main priorities in your routines. A more stable emotional state can be facilitated by consistency in these areas.
   - Form routines that promote mental health, such as journaling, practicing gratitude, or scheduling in time for introspection.

5. Open Communication: Encourage frank conversations about menopause with loved ones, family, and friends. The exchange of personal stories promotes empathy and establishes a nurturing atmosphere.
   - Normalize discussions about menopause to lessen stigma and promote candid discussion about the difficulties and successes of this stage of life.

6. Educate Yourself:Learn about menopause to gain a better understanding of the mental and physical changes that come with it.
   - Knowledge may allay anxieties of the unknown and give people the power to make decisions about their health and well-being.

7. Connect with Others:Attend in-person or online support groups where women going through menopause can talk about their experiences.

- Developing relationships with people who are aware of the difficulties helps foster a sense of belonging and lessen feelings of loneliness.

8. Seek Professional Guidance: If emotional difficulties continue, think about consulting therapists or counselors who specialize in mental health.
   - Expert assistance can offer coping mechanisms, a secure environment for communication, and direction on handling difficult emotions.

Rncouraging Open Communication and Seeking Assistance:

1. Normalize Conversations: Promote candid and open dialogue on menopause to dispel social stigmas and promote understanding.
   Normalize menopause experiences to foster an atmosphere where people are at ease sharing their struggles and looking for assistance.

2. Educate Others:– To debunk rumors and misconceptions, educate friends, family, and coworkers about menopause.
   - Greater empathy and support from people around you can result from increased awareness.

3. Express Your Needs: Make sure your loved ones are aware of what you require. Expressing your requirements creates a network of support, whether it's asking for help with everyday chores, understanding during trying times, or emotional support.

4. Promote Empathy:- Promote empathy by the sharing of individual experiences and feelings. This can lessen judgment and promote connection by generating a more sympathetic and understanding atmosphere.

5. Utilize Resources: - Make use of the resources that are accessible, such as educational publications, online forums, and medical specialists who specialize in menopause. Using resources can offer insightful information and assistance in overcoming obstacles.

6. Seek Professional Help: Do not be afraid to get professional assistance if emotional difficulties become too much to handle. Professionals in mental health can provide individualized counseling and assistance.

To sum up, coping strategy adoption, encouraging open communication, and seeking assistance are essential components of managing the emotional difficulties associated with menopause. Through the cultivation of a supportive environment on a personal and communal level, people can effectively manage this era of transition with resilience, empathy, and a sense of empowerment.

Dietary Guidelines for Menopause: Fueling Your Body During Transition

During menopause, which is a major life period that involves many bodily changes, maintaining a healthy, nutrient-rich diet is essential to promoting overall well-being. Nutritional decisions are critical for symptom management, bone health support, and emotional resilience building. The following food recommendations are specific to menopausal women and their needs:

1. Make Nutrient-Rich Foods a Priority: Make fruit, vegetables, whole grains, lean protein, and healthy fats the main components of your diet. These meals supply vital vitamins and minerals required for good general health.

2. Vitamin D and Calcium for Healthy Bones: Hormonal shifts during menopause may impact bone density. Make sure you're getting enough calcium and vitamin D to maintain healthy bones. Good sources include dairy products, fatty fish, leafy greens, and fortified cereals.

3. Omega-3 Fatty Acids for Heart Health:
Incorporate omega-3 fatty acid sources such as
walnuts, flaxseeds, chia seeds, and fatty fish
(salmon, mackerel). These heart-healthy fats also
have the potential to reduce hot flashes and other
related symptoms.

4. Protein-Rich Foods: Give lean meats, chicken,
fish, beans, lentils, and tofu the priority when it
comes to your diet. During menopause, protein
helps maintain a healthy weight and promotes the
health of muscles.
5
. Foods High in Phytoestrogen: Include foods high
in phytoestrogens, like whole grains, flaxseeds, and
soy products (tofu, edamame). Phytoestrogens
might provide a natural method of controlling
hormone swings.

6. Hydration is Key: Make sure you're getting
enough water throughout the day. Maintaining
adequate water promotes general health, aids with
weight management, and may ease symptoms like
hot flashes.
7. Minimize Alcohol and Caffeine: Consuming too
much alcohol or caffeine can aggravate symptoms
like hot flashes and cause sleep disturbances.

Reducing the use of these substances can improve general well-being.

8. Moderate Sugar Intake: Cut back on the amount of additional sugar you eat. Choose naturally occurring sweeteners like fruits to help you keep your weight in check and sustain steady energy levels.

9. Fiber for Digestive Health: To promote digestive health, eat a diet high in whole grains, fruits, vegetables, and legumes. Additionally, fiber helps to balance blood sugar levels and maintain weight.

10. Keep an eye on your sodium intake: Watch how much sodium you eat to help maintain heart health. Select complete foods that have undergone minimum processing, and use herbs and spices rather than a lot of salt to add taste.

11. consider Supplements: Speak with medical experts to ascertain whether supplements are required. Depending on a person's needs, supplements with omega-3 fatty acids, calcium, and vitamin D may be suggested.

12. Customize to Meet Specific Needs: Individual needs and preferences should guide nutritional

decisions throughout menopause because menopausal experiences differ. Pay attention to your body's signals and make changes in response to how particular foods affect your health.

Including these dietary recommendations in your routine may help control menopausal symptoms and improve general health. Always seek the advice of medical specialists for individualized guidance tailored to your unique needs and health profile. During this life-changing phase, feeding your body healthful meals is a potent method to boost your well-being.

Dietary Considerations: Examine how diet may help with symptom management

Dietary Considerations: Nourishing Your Body Through Change for Menopausal Symptom Management

A person's diet has a significant impact on managing the physical and emotional changes associated with menopause as well as enhancing overall wellbeing. Menopausal women can successfully support their bodies and address specific issues by eating a diet rich in nutrients and well-balanced.

1 Hot Flashes: Include foods high in phytoestrogens, like whole grains, flaxseeds, and soy products (tofu, edamame). Hot flashes are linked to hormonal variations that phytoestrogens may help control.
   - Steer clear of hot flash trigger foods, such as those high in caffeine, alcohol, or spice.

2. Bone Health: Make sure you're getting enough calcium and vitamin D to maintain the health of your bones. Good sources include dairy products, fatty fish, leafy greens, and fortified cereals.
   - Incorporate foods high in magnesium, which supports healthy muscles and bone density, such as nuts, seeds, and whole grains.

3. Variations in Mood and Anger:
   Give priority to the omega-3 fatty acids that can be found in walnuts, flaxseeds, chia seeds, and fatty fish. These beneficial fats may have a positive effect on mood and promote brain health.
   - Include complex carbs, such as whole grains and legumes, as these can help stabilize mood and blood sugar levels.

4. Sleep Disturbances: Reducing coffee and alcohol use, particularly in the evening, will help you get a better night's sleep.

   - Incorporate foods that promote sleep, such as healthy grains, cherries, and bananas, into your evening meals.

5. Weight Management: To promote general health and control weight, concentrate on eating a well-balanced diet that includes a range of nutrient-dense foods.

   Incorporate foods high in fiber, such as whole grains, fruits, and vegetables, as these support healthy digestion and satiety.

6 Vaginal Dryness: Eat more foods high in omega-7 fatty acids, like macadamia nuts and sea buckthorn berries, as these may help maintain the health of the mucous membranes.

   - Drink lots of water to stay hydrated; this is important for overall health, including hydration of mucous membranes.

7. Cognitive Changes: To promote brain health, give antioxidant-rich meals like berries, dark leafy greens, and almonds the priority.

- Incorporate meals rich in B vitamins, which are important for cognitive function and may be found in whole grains and leafy greens.

8. Emotional Welfare: Assure sufficient consumption of amino acids from foods high in protein, which will aid in the synthesis of neurotransmitters that affect mood.
  - Incorporate foods that improve mood, such as dark chocolate, which has precursors of serotonin.

9. Soreness in the joints and muscles:
  - Place a focus on foods that reduce inflammation, such as almonds, fatty salmon, and vibrant fruits and vegetables.
  - Maintain your fluid intake to promote flexibility and joint health.

10. Hydration and Overall Health: Make it a priority to be properly hydrated by sipping water all day long. Dehydration can affect general health and make several symptoms worse.
  Incorporate an array of vibrant fruits and vegetables to guarantee a wide range of nutrients.

Keep in mind that dietary recommendations should be tailored to each person's interests, health, and reactions to specific foods. Seeking advice from medical specialists, such as certified dietitians, can offer customized recommendations for controlling menopausal symptoms with food selections. During this life-changing phase, a comprehensive and thoughtful approach to nutrition can greatly support symptom management and general vitality.

Benefits of Diet Supplementation: Optimising Nutritious Consumption During Menopause

Dietary supplements, which target particular nutritional requirements, can be a useful addition to help those going through menopause. A varied and well-balanced diet is still essential, although supplements can provide certain advantages. Adding food supplements to your regimen during menopause has the following benefits:

1. Combining Missing Nutrients: - It might be difficult for postmenopausal women to get all the nutrients they need from food alone. Potential nutrient gaps can be filled with supplements, guaranteeing a sufficient intake of vitamins and minerals that are essential for general health.

2. Support for Bone Health:Supplements containing calcium and vitamin D may be especially helpful in maintaining bone health throughout menopause. As hormonal fluctuations may affect bone density, these nutrients become even more important.

3. Omega-3 Fatty Acids for Heart and Brain Health:Fish oil or algae-based omega-3 supplements can enhance cognitive performance and promote heart health. During menopause, these good fats are crucial for preserving general well-being.

4. Phytoestrogen Supplements:Plants like red clover and soy contain phytoestrogens, which act as the body's equivalent of estrogen. Hot flashes and other symptoms related to hormonal fluctuations may be lessened with the use of supplements containing phytoestrogens.

5. Vitamin B Complex: B vitamins are essential for both cognitive function and energy metabolism. Support may be provided by a B-complex supplement, particularly in cases where food intake is inadequate.

6. Iron and Vitamin C:If iron deficiency anemia is a possibility for some menopausal women, taking iron and vitamin C supplements may be beneficial. Iron absorption is improved by vitamin C, which supports energy levels generally.

7. Collagen Supplements for Skin Health:-During menopause, collagen levels, a protein essential for skin suppleness, may decrease. Collagen supplements can help hydrate and maintain the condition of the skin, addressing issues with dryness and aging.

8. Multivitamins:Supplements containing multiple vitamins offer a practical approach to ensure adequate intake of a wide range of vital nutrients. They provide a thorough method for promoting general health throughout menopause.

Well-Balanced Menopausal Diet: Fueling Your Body with Vital Nutrients

Supplements can be helpful, but they should be used in conjunction with a diet rich in nutrients and well-rounded. This is a well-balanced eating plan designed to meet the unique requirements of women going through menopause:

Rich in fiber, vitamins, and antioxidants, this whole-grain cereal with berries is a great choice for breakfast.
Greek Yogurt with Nuts & Seeds: Offers vital minerals, protein, and good fats.
Green Tea:May aid in metabolism and contains antioxidants.

Snack for Mid-Morning:Cubed Apple with Almond Butter:a blend of vitamins, fiber, and good fats.

Lunch:Grilled Salmon Salad: High in omega-3 fatty acids, colorful veggies, and leafy greens.
Brown rice or Quinoa: A good source of extra nutrients and complex carbohydrates.

Snack for the afternoon: Carrot sticks with hummus: A filling and healthy choice.

Supper:- Grilled Tofu or Chicken Breast:bOffers lean protein.
Steamed Sweet Potato with Broccoli: Packed with nutrients and vitamins.
Olive Oil Dressing: Provides a boost of good fats.

Evening Snack: Cabotage cheese mixed with berries: provides a blend of antioxidants and protein.

Hydration: cucumber or Lemon Infused Water:
Drink plenty of water throughout the day.

Supplementary Considerations: Supplementary
Calcium and Vitamin D:in case of inadequate food
intake.
Omega-3 Fatty Acid Supplement:Particularly for
people who don't eat a lot of seafood.
Multivitamin with B-Complex: To guarantee a
thorough consumption of vital elements.

Talk to Medical Professionals:
It's important to speak with medical specialists
before taking supplements to determine your
specific nutritional needs and any possible drug
interactions. Personalized advice might be given by
them based on certain health profiles.

To sum up:
Optimizing nutritional intake during menopause
can be achieved through a combination of a
well-balanced food plan and prudent supplement
use. During this pivotal time of life, making dietary
decisions based on personal needs, taking
supplements into account when needed, and
consulting medical professionals are all important
for overall well-being.

Recognize how supplements help maintain hormonal balance

Appropriate Supplementation: Preserving Hormonal Equilibrium

It is impossible to overestimate the importance of vitamins in preserving hormonal balance when it comes to general health. Hormones are essential for controlling a wide range of biological processes, including mood, energy levels, metabolism, and more. Hormonal changes brought on by aging, especially in women going through menopause, can cause a variety of symptoms. Appropriate supplementation becomes an important tactic to assist with hormonal balance and advance ideal health.

Comprehending the complex interactions of hormones is crucial. Hormones function as intermediaries, facilitating communication among various bodily functions and systems. Mood fluctuations, weariness, weight gain, and sleep difficulties are just a few symptoms that can arise from changes in this delicate equilibrium. Here's where thoughtful supplements can have a big impact.

A sensible approach to augmenting involves appreciating the significance of a comprehensive strategy. An all-encompassing approach that includes a balanced diet, consistent exercise, and stress management is crucial rather than depending just on individual supplements. Nonetheless, some nutrients may be very helpful in treating hormonal abnormalities.

The synthesis and operation of hormones depend heavily on vitamins and minerals. For example, minerals like zinc and magnesium are involved in different hormonal processes, while vitamin D is believed to support the generation of sex hormones. Including a wide variety of meals high in nutrients and, if required, supplements can help to keep these vital components at their ideal levels.

Fish oil and flaxseed, which contain omega-3 fatty acids, are two other supplement classes that are worth looking into. These fats are involved in hormonal balance, especially when it comes to lowering inflammation and promoting mental wellness. By including omega-3 pills in their routine, women going through menopause may experience relief from joint pain and mood changes.

Hormonal abnormalities, particularly during menopause, have traditionally been treated with herbal remedies, such as evening primrose oil and black cohosh. Although there is still much to learn about their efficacy in science, many women say they feel better when it comes to problems like mood swings and hot flashes.

It's important to proceed cautiously when using supplements and to speak with medical professionals before implementing any big regular adjustments. Since everyone's demands are different, a tailored approach guarantees that supplements are selected by particular health objectives and specifications.

In conclusion, maintaining hormonal balance with prudent supplementation is a complex process. It entails understanding the complex relationships that exist between lifestyle, hormone health, and diet. People can help their bodies navigate the changes that come with aging by including a wide variety of minerals, important fatty acids, and properly selected herbal supplements, which will enhance general health and vitality.

Emphasize the need of essential vitamins and minerals for menopausal women

Stressing Menopausal Women's Need for Vital Vitamins and Minerals

For women, menopause is a major life transition that is followed by hormonal changes that may affect general health and well-being. Important vitamins and minerals are needed at this phase to help the body overcome the special difficulties caused by changes in hormone levels. Promoting menopausal women's optimal health requires an understanding of the roles played by particular nutrients and making sure they are consumed in sufficient amounts.

1. Density and Calcium:

The increased risk of osteoporosis and bone density loss following menopause is one of the main causes of concern. Vitamin D and calcium are very important for keeping strong bones. To achieve their calcium demands, menopausal women should give priority to dairy products, leafy green vegetables, and fortified meals. Calcium absorption is aided by vitamin D, which is commonly produced by exposure to sunlight and can be supplemented if needed.

2. Complex B Vitamin

The B-vitamin family, which includes folate, B6, and B12, is critical for maintaining hormonal balance and general health. These vitamins aid in the metabolism of energy, maintain mental clarity and lessen the symptoms of menopause, including weariness and mood swings. Lean proteins, leafy greens, and whole grains all help to ensure that these essential nutrients are consumed in sufficient amounts.

3. Fatty Acids Omega

Cardiovascular issues are common among menopausal women. Walnuts, flaxseeds, and fatty fish are good sources of omega-3 fatty acids, which are essential for heart health. These good fats may help lower inflammation, control cholesterol levels, and possibly even aid with hot flashes and other related symptoms.

4. Egg:

Vitamin E, which is well-known for having antioxidant qualities, may help with some menopausal symptoms. Vitamin E, which is present in nuts, seeds, and vegetable oils, has been linked to a decrease in hot flashes and may support skin health at this time of life.

5. Magnesium:

Magnesium has a role in several body processes, such as bone health, blood glucose regulation, and muscle and neuron function. Foods high in magnesium, such as leafy greens, nuts, and whole grains, may be beneficial to menopausal women because magnesium supplementation has been associated with better sleep and less anxiety.

6. Iron:

Menopausal women still need to consume enough iron, but because they are no longer menstruating, their needs are lower after menopause. For the blood to carry oxygen and for general energy levels, iron is essential. Lean meats, legumes, and fortified cereals can all be included to help you reach your iron goals.

7. Calcium

Vitamin C is essential for the production of collagen, healthy skin, and a strong immune system. Bell peppers, berries, and citrus fruits are good additions to a menopausal woman's diet to help with these vital processes.

In conclusion, addressing the physical and emotional changes related to this stage of life requires highlighting the importance of vitamins and minerals for menopausal women. A nutrient-dense, well-balanced diet, together with thoughtful supplementation when needed, can help women face menopause with resilience and support their long-term health and vitality. Seeking individualized guidance from healthcare specialists guarantees that requirements are addressed, promoting a comprehensive approach to well-being throughout this moment of transition.

Stress the need of speaking with medical specialists for specific guidance

Emphasizing the Need for Consulting Medical Experts for Specific Advice

Consultation with medical specialists is crucial when it comes to health issues, especially during major life transitions like menopause. Although broad knowledge and lifestyle modifications can serve as a basis for well-being, each person's health is distinct and necessitates tailored guidance. Seeking advice from medical experts guarantees a thorough comprehension of one's unique requirements, potential hazards, and advantages for the best possible care of one's health.

1. Personalized Evaluation:

Each woman's menopausal experience is unique and impacted by her lifestyle, general health, and heredity. Medical professionals with specialized training, such as endocrinologists and gynecologists, are qualified to provide customized evaluations. These evaluations consider the medical background, current health issues, and particular menopausal symptoms of the woman. This customized method enables the discovery of individualized approaches to deal with particular problems.

2. Hormonal Balancing and Available Therapies:

Menopause is characterized by hormone fluctuations, which frequently result in symptoms that affect day-to-day functioning. Health professionals can measure hormone levels and talk about possible therapies, such as hormone replacement therapy (HRT). Although some women benefit from HRT, it's important to weigh the dangers and advantages according to each person's unique health profile. Healthcare providers assist people in making well-informed decisions regarding their health by guiding them through these factors.

3. Control of Symptom Alleviation:

Menopausal symptoms can include mood fluctuations, weight gain, sleep problems, and hot flashes. A major part of managing symptom relief is the involvement of medical specialists. Depending on the needs of the patient, they may prescribe medicine, offer alternative therapy, or advise lifestyle modifications. This focused strategy raises the overall quality of life during menopause and increases the efficacy of therapies.

4. Orthoporosis Prevention and Bone Health:

Osteoporosis and bone fractures are more common in postmenopausal women. To prevent or manage osteoporosis, medical professionals, especially rheumatologists and bone health specialists, can measure bone density, offer dietary advice, and suggest the right supplements. Long-term skeletal health is protected in large part by this preventive measure.

5. Evaluation of Cardiovascular Health:

Because menopause is linked to changes in cardiovascular health, it's critical to identify and control any risks. Cardiologists can assess heart health, suggest lifestyle changes, and talk about the right drugs to reduce cardiovascular risks at this point in life. This all-encompassing strategy guarantees that women obtain focused advice to support heart health and general well-being.

6. Mental and Emotional Assistance:

Emotional and mental health can be affected by menopausal changes. The provision of assistance and coping mechanisms for the psychological elements of menopause is an area of expertise for psychologists and mental health practitioners. Consulting with these experts can help with anxiety and mood swings as well as build mental toughness and emotional health.

7. Regular Health Examinations:

For women both during and after menopause, routine health screenings including mammograms, Pap smears, and bone density testing are still essential. Based on each patient's unique risk factors, medical specialists organize these tests to ensure prompt identification and treatment of any possible health problems.

To sum up, it is critical to emphasize that seeking specific advice from medical professionals is essential to navigating menopause with proactive health management and informed decision-making. While broad guidance might serve as a starting point, the specialized insights offered by experts enable women to adopt a customized approach to their health, promoting resilience and well-being throughout this pivotal time of life.

Chapter 4

Menopause and Fitness

Menopause and Fitness: Using Exercise to Help with the Transition

Hormonal shifts that cause both physical and emotional changes are what define menopause, a normal and unavoidable stage in a woman's life. Being physically active regularly becomes essential to overcoming the obstacles that arise with menopause. In addition to aiding with symptom management, exercise improves general health by fostering bone density, cardiovascular health, and mental toughness throughout this time of change.

1. Controlling Body Mass and Metabolism:

Hormonal changes during menopause can cause weight gain and a change in the makeup of the body in women. Frequent exercise is essential for controlling weight since it increases metabolism and maintains lean muscle mass. Maintaining a healthy body weight and composition can be achieved by combining strength training, flexibility training, and cardiovascular activity.

2. Strength Training and Bone Health:

Women who have gone through menopause are more susceptible to osteoporosis, which highlights the need to engage in activities that promote bone health. Weight-bearing exercises and other strength training improve bone density and lower the risk of fractures. Long-term skeletal health is promoted by weightlifting, resistance training, and physical activities such as dancing that help to develop and maintain bone strength.

3. Cardiovascular Health:

Changes in cardiovascular health, including a higher risk of heart disease, are linked to menopause. Frequent cardiovascular activity, which includes cycling, swimming, running, and brisk walking, improves circulation, lowers blood pressure, and controls cholesterol levels, all of which contribute to the maintenance of heart health. These advantages lower the risk of cardiovascular illnesses and enhance overall cardiovascular resistance.

4. Managing the Symptoms of Menopause:

Hot flashes, mood swings, and sleep difficulties
are just a few of the menopausal symptoms that
exercise has been demonstrated to reduce.
Engaging in aerobic exercises triggers the release of
endorphins, which elevate mood and lessen stress.
Relaxation techniques like yoga and tai chi can help
manage stress even more and improve the quality
of your sleep.

5. Hormonal Equilibrium:

Exercise helps improve hormonal balance and
lessen related symptoms, but it cannot reverse the
hormonal changes brought on by menopause.
Exercise promotes hormonal balance, lowers
insulin resistance, and helps control cortisol levels.
Consequently, this leads to elevated mood,
increased vitality, and an all-around feeling of
well-being.

6. Health and Flexibility of the Joints:

Women going through menopause may notice
joint stiffness and decreased flexibility. Frequent
stretches and yoga poses improve flexibility and

joint mobility, which lowers the chance of injury and increases general physical comfort. Incorporating diverse stretches into the workout regimen promotes joint well-being and alleviates pain connected to age-related alterations.

7. The Mind-Body Link:

Menopause involves emotional and mental changes in addition to physical ones. Women can establish a positive mind-body connection through exercise by connecting with their bodies. During this transitional stage, engaging in mindful practices like as meditation or mind-body workshops helps with stress management, emotional stability, and a greater sense of control.

To sum up, the correlation between menopause and physical fitness highlights the need for consistent physical exercise to enhance general health and wellness. Women can embrace the good effects of an active lifestyle on their physical and emotional well-being and traverse menopause with resilience by implementing a well-rounded exercise regimen that incorporates cardiovascular fitness, strength training, flexibility, and stress management. It can be helpful to customize an exercise program to meet the needs of each individual, working with healthcare professionals or fitness specialists to ensure a safe and efficient way to stay active during this important stage of life.

Exercise Methods: Adapting Exercise Programs for Women Affected by Menopause

Adapting exercise practices is essential as women go through menopause to handle the special opportunities and challenges brought on by hormonal changes. Adapting exercise routines to menopause-related symptoms can improve general health and the efficacy of exercise programs. Women can adapt their workout routines to get through this transitional time with resilience and comfort by adding certain tactics.

1. Consideration for Cardiovascular Exercise:

There is a strong correlation between menopause and alterations in heart health. Cardiovascular activity should not be neglected, but comfort should always come first. Low-impact exercises that don't overly stress joints, like swimming, cycling, or brisk walking, can improve cardiovascular health. Combining short bursts of intense activity with longer rest intervals is known as interval training, and it is beneficial for both weight management and heart health.

2. Strength Exercise for Healthy Bones:

Following menopause, bone density tends to decline, raising the risk of osteoporosis. Weight-bearing workouts and other strength training are essential for maintaining bone health. Including resistance training with weight machines, resistance bands, or free weights promotes and preserves bone density. To increase general strength and stability, concentrate on the main muscular groups in your body, such as your arms, legs, hips, and back.

3. Joint health and flexibility:

Women going through menopause may notice joint stiffness and decreased flexibility. It's essential to incorporate stretching exercises into the regimen to improve joint mobility and lower the chance of injury. Exercises that focus on balance and flexibility, like yoga or Pilates, might be very helpful. Main muscle groups should be gently stretched to preserve flexibility and enhance joint health in general.

4. Intentional Training Techniques:

Menopause involves emotional and mental changes in addition to physical ones. Exercises that require mindfulness, like tai chi or yoga, can have a twofold effect by enhancing physical and mental health. During this transitional moment, these mind-body activities support women in managing stress, enhancing general mental resilience, and improving mood.

5. Practical Training for Everyday Tasks:

Women who incorporate functional exercises into their program are better able to maintain their strength and agility for daily tasks. Functional training imitates everyday motions including bending, lifting, and squatting. This method not only increases general fitness but also makes it easier to carry out daily duties.

6. Moderating Duration and Intensity:

Exercise tolerance may be impacted by menopausal symptoms such as hot flashes and exhaustion. Ladies should pay attention to their bodies and be willing to modify the length and intensity of their workouts. Frequent, shorter sessions could be more productive and well-tolerated. Choosing to work out indoors or during cooler hours of the day can also assist in controlling discomfort caused by temperature.

7. Control of Temperature and Hydration:

The control of body temperature may alter in women going through menopause. It's crucial to stay hydrated, especially when exercising. Overheating can be controlled by exercising in well-ventilated areas and dressing breathable. A comfortable and long-lasting exercise regimen is facilitated by maintaining one's own pace and scheduling breaks as necessary.

8. Healthcare Professional Consultation:

Menopausal women should speak with medical doctors or fitness specialists before starting or changing an exercise program. Exercise suggestions can be more specifically tailored when a thorough evaluation of each person's health is performed, taking into account current medical problems and drug use. This guarantees a menopausal exercise regimen that is both safe and successful.

In summary, modifying exercise regimens for women experiencing menopause necessitates a careful and customized strategy. Women can address the mental and physical aspects of this time of life by combining mindfulness techniques, aerobic exercise, strength training, and flexibility exercises. Tailoring workouts to the specific requirements and preferences of menopausal women encourages a good exercise experience, which in turn fosters resilience and general well-being during this life-changing stage.

Stress the importance of exercise in symptom management

Emphasizing the Value of Physical Activity in Symptom Management

Frequent exercise turns out to be an effective tool for addressing a wide range of symptoms linked to different medical disorders, including menopause. Hormonal changes brought on by the transformational phase of menopause can cause a variety of symptoms, including mood swings, hot flashes, insomnia, and weight gain. It becomes imperative to emphasize the role exercise plays in symptom management to provide women with a proactive, all-encompassing strategy for overcoming the obstacles associated with this life transition.

1. Reducing Night Sweats and Hot Flashes:

Night sweats and hot flashes are two of the most prevalent and bothersome menopausal symptoms. Regular aerobic exercise has been demonstrated to lessen these episodes' frequency and intensity. Exercises that improve cardiovascular health overall, such as brisk walking, cycling, or swimming, can help control body temperature and possibly lessen the frequency of hot flashes. Consistently engaging in physical activity also helps to improve general sleep patterns, alleviate night sweats, and improve the quality of sleep.

2. Detoxification and Mood Improvement:

Women going through menopause frequently have mood fluctuations, impatience, and elevated stress levels. Exercise releases endorphins, which are feel-good hormones that promote well-being and act as a natural mood enhancer. Including

exercises like yoga, dance, or jogging in the regimen
gives people an outlet for their emotions, lowers
stress levels, and strengthens their mental
toughness. The general quality of life during
menopause can be greatly enhanced by the
beneficial effects of exercise on mood.

3. Metabolic Health and Weight Management:

Weight gain and a change in body composition
can be attributed to hormonal changes that occur
during the menopause. Frequent exercise is
essential for maintaining metabolic health and
controlling weight. Strength training and
cardiovascular exercise together help you keep a
healthy weight, burn calories, and maintain lean
muscle mass. Consequently, this lowers the
likelihood of health problems associated with
obesity and enhances general metabolic health.

4. Improving the Health of Bones:

An increased risk of osteoporosis and bone
fractures is linked to the decrease in estrogen levels
that occurs following menopause. Strength training
and weightlifting are essential elements of an
exercise program that promotes bone health. These
exercises improve bone density, promote bone

remodeling, and lower the incidence of fractures, all of which are beneficial to menopausal women's long-term skeletal health.

5. Enhancing the Quality of Sleep:

During menopause, sleep disruptions are prevalent and are frequently made worse by symptoms connected to hormone imbalances. Frequent exercise has a beneficial effect on sleep patterns, particularly when done early in the day. It lowers anxiety, encourages relaxation, and aids in the regulation of circadian cycles, all of which enhance the quality of sleep. One of the most effective ways to treat menopausal sleep difficulties is to establish a regular exercise regimen.

6. Improving Heart and Circulatory Health:

Cardiovascular health changes with menopause, including a higher risk of heart disease. Regular cardiovascular activity lowers blood pressure, regulates cholesterol, and improves circulation, all of which are factors that support heart health. To lower the risk of cardiovascular illnesses both during and after menopause, these advantages are crucial.

7. Brain Health and Cognitive Function:

Menopause-related hormonal changes can affect cognitive function; some women experience memory loss and concentration issues. It has been demonstrated that exercise improves brain function and neuroplasticity, which in turn benefits cognition. In particular, aerobic exercises enhance blood flow to the brain, promoting cognitive health and possibly mitigating cognitive problems associated with menopause.

In summary, emphasizing the role that exercise plays in helping menopausal women manage their symptoms is a comprehensive strategy for improving general well-being. Frequent exercise not only helps with particular symptoms but also builds mental and emotional toughness throughout this transitional stage. Women who are encouraged to adopt a varied and pleasurable exercise regimen that suits their requirements and preferences are better equipped to manage the symptoms of menopause and take an active and positive approach to this important life transition.

A key component of overall health is hormonal balance, which is even more crucial during important life stages like menopause. Exercises for strength and flexibility shown to be effective means of preserving hormonal balance, providing a comprehensive strategy that goes beyond physical fitness to favorably influence hormonal health. The relationship that exists between exercise, hormones, and overall health emphasizes how important it is to include strength and flexibility exercises in one's routine.

1. The Effect of Strength Training on Hormones:

Exercises for strengthening the muscles with weights, resistance bands, or body weight are referred to as resistance or weight training. This type of physical activity triggers the release of hormones that support the development of muscle, control metabolism, and maintain hormonal equilibrium. For example, resistance training has been linked to higher levels of testosterone and growth hormone production, two essential substances for preserving bone density, muscular mass, and metabolic processes.

2. Hormonal balance and metabolic health:

Hormonal abnormalities can cause metabolic problems that affect how well people manage their weight and feel overall. Strength training increases muscular mass, which improves the body's capacity to burn calories effectively and regulates metabolism. This increase in metabolism has a beneficial effect on insulin sensitivity, assisting in blood sugar regulation and lowering the risk of metabolic diseases. Strength training supports a balanced metabolic state, which is beneficial for hormone balance and overall health.

3. Hormone-Related and Bone Health Benefits:

Women are more prone to osteoporosis due to the decrease in estrogen that occurs following menopause, which puts their bone health in danger. Exercises involving weight bearing, specifically strength training, act as a preventative measure against the loss of bone density. The body releases growth hormone and insulin-like growth factor (IGF-1) in response to resistance in the bones, which increases bone density. The beneficial effects on bone health are consistent with the overarching objective of preserving hormonal balance during the menopausal transition.

4. Exercises for Flexibility and the Reduction of Stress Hormones:

Exercises that improve flexibility, such as yoga and stretching techniques, are essential for managing stress. Prolonged stress can raise cortisol levels, which can upset hormonal balance and be a factor in several health problems. Including flexibility exercises in the regimen has been shown to lower cortisol levels, improve relaxation, and ease muscle tension. Flexibility exercises help to maintain hormonal equilibrium and promote emotional well-being during menopause by reducing stress hormone reactions.

5. Endorphin Production and Control of Mood:

Exercises for strength and flexibility both help the body's natural mood enhancers, endorphins, to be released. As neurotransmitters, endorphins work with brain receptors to lessen pain perception and increase emotions of well-being. This effect on mood regulation is especially important during menopause, as changes in hormones can have an impact on mental health. Frequent strength and

flexibility training is a natural, all-encompassing
method of treating mood-related symptoms
brought on by hormone fluctuations.

6. Enhanced Sensitivity to Insulin:

Insulin sensitivity, a critical component of
hormonal homeostasis, has been demonstrated to
be improved by strength training. Increased
sensitivity to insulin enables cells to react to it more
effectively, resulting in a more effective uptake of
glucose. This promotes general hormonal balance
by assisting in the regulation of hormone levels,
especially insulin, and promoting metabolic health.

7. A Comprehensive Approach to Hormonal Health:

Exercises for flexibility and strength combined
have a holistic effect on hormone health. Flexibility
exercises help to reduce stress and regulate mood,
while strength training targets the health of muscles
and bones and influences the synthesis of growth
hormone and testosterone. Combining the two
kinds of exercise into a well-rounded program
improves the hormonal milieu overall, which
fosters health and vitality.

Conclusively, stressing the importance of strength and flexibility training in preserving hormonal equilibrium is a proactive and powerful strategy, particularly in life phases such as menopause. Through deliberate integration of these activities into a daily regimen, people can enhance hormone levels, promoting mental, physical, and metabolic health. This all-encompassing viewpoint emphasizes how exercise and hormone health are linked, enabling people to go through life's changes with resiliency and vitality.

Chapter 5

Menopause and Sleep: Recognizing the Effects and Developing Better Strategies

Menopause is a natural stage that occurs as a woman's reproductive years come to an end. It is accompanied by major hormonal changes that can have a substantial impact on sleep patterns and overall quality of sleep. Women frequently have sleep difficulties during this phase, including insomnia, sweating during the night, and changes in their sleep patterns. It's critical to comprehend how menopause affects sleep and put improvement techniques into practice to support general well-being during this life-changing stage.

1. Disturbances in Hormones and Sleep:

The reduction in estrogen and progesterone levels, in particular, is a major factor in sleep problems following menopause. As women approach menopause, estrogen levels decrease, which causes disturbances in sleep patterns.

Estrogen is believed to control the sleep-wake cycle and promote deep sleep. The sedative hormone progesterone also declines, which exacerbates sleep problems. Furthermore, changes in other hormones like melatonin and cortisol can affect the quantity and quality of sleep.

2. Typical Sleep Problems During Menopause:

Menopausal women frequently encounter a variety of sleep disorders, such as:

- Insomnia: The inability to fall or keep asleep through the night.
- Hot flashes and night sweats: Abrupt bursts of extreme heat and perspiration that frequently interfere with sleep.
- Sleep fragmentation: Recurring awakenings during the night cause the architecture of sleep to be disturbed.
- Mood-related sleep disturbances: The length and quality of sleep can be impacted by anxiety, anger, and mood changes.
- Restless legs syndrome: Uncomfortable sensations in the legs that frequently result in a strong need to move them, which keeps people awake at night.

3. Implications for General Health and Welfare:

Sleep problems have more negative effects on general health and well-being than just exhaustion. Menopause-related chronic sleep deprivation has been linked to higher risk factors for metabolic diseases, mental disorders, cardiovascular disease, and cognitive impairment. Therefore, addressing sleep problems is essential to reducing these risks and enhancing general health and vigor throughout menopause.

4. Tips for Enhancing Sleep Throughout Menopause:

Menopause-related sleep problems can be difficult to manage, but several techniques can help increase the quantity and quality of sleep:

- Creating a regular sleep schedule: The body's internal clock is regulated and improved sleep is encouraged when bed and wake times are fixed for each day.
- Establishing a sleep-friendly environment: Make sure the bedroom is cool, quiet, and dark, with cozy bedding and few outside distractions.
- Managing stress: Relaxation methods like deep breathing, yoga, or meditation might help you sleep

better because stress can make sleep problems worse.

- Including consistent exercise: Regular physical activity can help balance hormones and enhance the quality of sleep, especially early in the day.

- Nutritional factors: Better sleep can be supported by avoiding stimulants like caffeine and alcohol close to bedtime and choosing foods that promote sleep, such as lean proteins, complex carbs, and foods high in magnesium.

- Seeking medical advice: Speaking with medical professionals, such as gynecologists or sleep specialists, can offer tailored advice and solutions for treating sleep difficulties associated with menopause.

5. Sleep with Hormone Replacement Therapy (HRT):

Hormone replacement treatment (HRT) may be suggested for certain women to relieve menopausal symptoms, such as insomnia. In particular, estrogen therapy has been demonstrated to enhance the quality of sleep and lessen the frequency of hot flashes and night sweats in women going through menopause. On the other hand, deciding whether to pursue HRT should be done after consulting medical experts and considering the risks and advantages according to each person's unique health profile.

6. Insomnia Cognitive Behavior Therapy (CBT-I):

An organized program called cognitive-behavioral treatment for insomnia (CBT-I) aims to address the underlying causes of sleep problems. CBT-I focuses on changing the attitudes and behaviors that lead to insomnia, encouraging better sleeping practices, and enhancing the quality of sleep. It has been demonstrated that this evidence-based strategy works well for treating sleep difficulties brought on by menopause.

In conclusion, the hormonal shifts and accompanying symptoms of menopause can have a substantial impact on sleep quality and general well-being. To promote maximum health and energy at this life-changing moment, it is imperative to comprehend the variables that contribute to sleep problems and put improvement techniques into practice. Through lifestyle adjustments, relaxation methods, and medicinal interventions when required, women can manage sleep problems during menopause and embrace restorative sleep as essential to their overall health.

Understanding Sleep Disruptions

Comprehending Sleep Disruptions: Origins, Impacts, and Methods for Enhancement

Sleep disturbances are frequent and can have a serious negative effect on general health and well-being. Sleep disturbances can take many different forms, from trouble falling asleep to frequent nighttime awakenings. These can result in daytime tiredness, mood swings, and diminished cognitive function. Promoting restful sleep and optimum well-being requires an understanding of the underlying causes of sleep disruptions, their implications on health, and the application of therapeutic measures.

1. Reasons for Sleep Disorders:

Numerous things might cause sleep disturbances, such as:

- Stress and Anxiety: Psychological stressors can make it difficult to unwind and go to sleep, such as pressures from the workplace or interpersonal disputes.
- Bad Sleep Habits: Sleep patterns can be disturbed by irregular sleep schedules, excessive

screen time before bed, and the consumption of stimulants like caffeine or alcohol close to bedtime.

- Medical Conditions: Sleep quality can be greatly impacted by respiratory conditions like sleep apnea, psychological conditions like anxiety or depression, and chronic pain.

- Hormonal Changes: Sleep difficulties may result from fluctuations in hormone levels, which may occur during menstruation, pregnancy, or menopause.

- Environmental Factors: Uncomfortable bedding, light pollution, noise, and an inappropriate sleep environment can all make it difficult to have a good night's sleep.

2. Health Effects of Sleep Disruptions:

Sleep disturbances have more effects on one's physical, emotional, and cognitive well-being than just being tired.

- Impaired Cognitive Function: Sleep issues can lead to problems with focus, memory, and decision-making, which can have an impact on performance at work or in the classroom.

- Mood Disorders: Extended sleep deprivation is associated with elevated irritability, mood fluctuations, and signs of anxiety and despair.

- Weakened Immune Function: Not getting enough sleep weakens the immune system, making one more vulnerable to infections and prolonging the time it takes to recover from illness.
- Risks to Cardiovascular Health: Sleep disruptions are linked to a higher risk of heart disease, stroke, hypertension, and other cardiovascular disorders.
- Metabolic Disorders: Sleep deprivation throws off hormone balance, which raises the risk of obesity, diabetes, and metabolic syndrome as well as irregularities in hormones that control hunger.
- Decreased Quality of Life: Sleep disturbances that persist can have a major negative impact on relationships, productivity at work, and general well-being.

3. Tips for Increasing Sleep Quality:

To resolve sleep disturbances, one must establish healthy sleeping habits and address the underlying causes of poor sleep, which include:

- Create a regular sleep schedule: Maintaining a regular bedtime and wake-up time each day aids in regulating the body's internal clock and enhances the quality of sleep.

- Establish a sleeping-friendly environment: Make sure the bedroom has a supportive mattress, and pillows, and is quiet, dark, and cozy.

- Use relaxing methods: The body can become more relaxed and primed for sleep through deep breathing, mindfulness exercises, progressive muscular relaxation, and meditation.

- Limit electronics and stimulants right before bed: Steer clear of alcohol, nicotine, and caffeine right before bed, and limit your screen time to avoid blue light exposure, which can cause sleep disturbances.

- Control your stress: Before going to bed, try some stress-relieving exercises like yoga, tai chi, or journaling to release tension and encourage relaxation.

- Seek medical evaluation: Speak with a healthcare provider to see whether there are any underlying medical illnesses or sleep disorders and to discuss treatment options if sleep disturbances continue despite lifestyle changes.

4. Expert Sleep Disorder Interventions:

Professional interventions may be required for people who have severe or persistent sleep disturbances:

- Cognitive-behavioral treatment for insomnia (CBT-I): This systematic approach targets the root causes of insomnia and helps alter beliefs and behaviors that exacerbate sleep disturbances, encouraging better sleep hygiene and higher-quality sleep.

- Medical interventions: Continuous positive airway pressure (CPAP) therapy or medication may be recommended to treat sleep disorders including sleep apnea or restless legs syndrome to reduce symptoms and enhance the quality of sleep.

To sum up, comprehending sleep disturbances entails identifying the various elements that can affect the quality of sleep and putting tactics in place to encourage restorative sleep. Prioritizing restorative sleep can help people improve their general health and well-being by addressing underlying reasons, forming healthy sleep habits, and seeking appropriate interventions when necessary.

Examine typical menopausal sleep problems

Examination of Typical Menopausal Sleep Problems

Menopause, a natural phase marking the end of a woman's reproductive years, brings about significant hormonal changes that can profoundly impact sleep patterns and overall sleep quality. Sleep problems are prevalent during this transition, affecting a large proportion of menopausal women. Understanding the typical sleep problems experienced during menopause is essential for effective management and improvement of sleep quality during this transformative phase of life.

1. Insomnia:

Insomnia, characterized by difficulty falling asleep, staying asleep, or waking up too early and being unable to return to sleep, is a common sleep problem experienced by menopausal women. Hormonal fluctuations, particularly the decline in estrogen levels, can disrupt the body's natural sleep-wake cycle, leading to insomnia. Additionally, factors such as hot flashes, night sweats, and mood disturbances associated with menopause can exacerbate insomnia symptoms.

2. Hot Flashes and Night Sweats:

Hot flashes and night sweats are hallmark symptoms of menopause and can significantly disrupt sleep. These sudden episodes of intense heat and sweating can occur during the night, leading to night awakenings and difficulty returning to sleep. The body's temperature regulation mechanisms become dysregulated during menopause, contributing to the occurrence of hot flashes and night sweats, which can have a profound impact on sleep quality and duration.

3. Sleep Fragmentation:

Menopausal women often experience sleep fragmentation, characterized by frequent awakenings during the night. These interruptions in sleep continuity can disrupt the normal sleep architecture, leading to non-restorative sleep and daytime fatigue. Factors such as hormonal fluctuations, anxiety, and mood disturbances can contribute to sleep fragmentation during menopause, further exacerbating sleep problems.

4. Mood-related Sleep Disturbances:

Mood disturbances, including anxiety, irritability, and depression, are common during menopause and can significantly impact sleep quality. Women experiencing mood-related symptoms may find it difficult to relax and fall asleep, leading to insomnia. Additionally, mood disturbances can contribute to sleep fragmentation and disrupt the overall sleep-wake cycle, further exacerbating sleep problems during menopause.

5. Restless Legs Syndrome (RLS):

Restless legs syndrome (RLS) is characterized by uncomfortable sensations in the legs, often described as tingling, crawling, or itching sensations, accompanied by an irresistible urge to move the legs. RLS symptoms typically worsen at night and can interfere with the ability to fall asleep or stay asleep. While the exact cause of RLS is not fully understood, hormonal changes and alterations in dopamine levels during menopause may contribute to its onset or exacerbation.

6. Snoring and Sleep Apnea:

Snoring and sleep apnea, characterized by pauses in breathing during sleep, are more prevalent in menopausal women compared to premenopausal women. Hormonal changes, weight gain, and alterations in upper airway anatomy during menopause can increase the risk of snoring and sleep apnea. These sleep-disordered breathing patterns can lead to fragmented sleep, daytime fatigue, and an increased risk of cardiovascular and metabolic disorders if left untreated.

7. Shifts in Sleep Architecture:

Menopause is associated with changes in sleep architecture, including alterations in the distribution of sleep stages and reductions in overall sleep efficiency. Rapid eye movement (REM) sleep, which is critical for cognitive function and emotional processing, may be disrupted during menopause, leading to cognitive impairment and mood disturbances. These shifts in sleep architecture contribute to sleep problems experienced by menopausal women and can impact overall health and well-being.

In conclusion, typical sleep problems experienced during menopause encompass a range of symptoms, including insomnia, hot flashes, night sweats, sleep fragmentation, mood-related disturbances, restless legs syndrome, and sleep-disordered breathing patterns. Understanding the underlying causes and mechanisms contributing to these sleep problems is essential for effective management and improvement of sleep quality during menopause. By addressing hormonal fluctuations, implementing lifestyle modifications, and seeking appropriate interventions when needed, menopausal women can enhance sleep quality and promote overall health and well-being during this transformative phase of life.

Practical Tips to Improve the Quality of Your Sleep

Although many people have trouble getting deep, restful sleep, it is crucial for good health and well-being. Thankfully, several techniques and lifestyle modifications can encourage improved sleep hygiene and higher-quality sleep. You may improve the quality of your sleep and reap the many advantages of getting a good night's sleep by implementing these routines into your everyday life.

1. Make a Regular Sleep Schedule:

Keeping a consistent sleep-wake schedule is essential to maximizing the quality of your sleep. Even on the weekends, try to get to bed and wake up at the same time every day. Maintaining consistency aids in the regulation of your body's circadian rhythm, facilitating effortless sleep and wakefulness. A more restful sleep experience and a lower chance of sleep interruptions can both be achieved by avoiding significant shifts in sleep patterns.

2. Establish a Relaxing Sleep Environment:

A major factor in encouraging restful sleep is the environment in which you sleep. Make sure your bedroom is cold, quiet, and dark so that you can sleep well. Invest in pillows and a comfy mattress that will support your body well. To further drown out any distracting noises that can keep you up at night, think about utilizing white noise generators or earplugs.

3. Reduce Screen Time Before Bed:

Your body's normal cycle of sleep and wakefulness may be disrupted if you spend time in front of a screen before bed, including laptops, tablets, and smartphones. Melatonin, a hormone that controls sleep, is suppressed by the blue light that electronic devices emit. Set a digital curfew at least an hour before bed and substitute it with calming activities like reading, having a warm bath, or practicing relaxation techniques to encourage better sleep.

4. Employ Methods of Relaxation:

Deep breathing, meditation, and progressive muscle relaxation are examples of relaxation practices that can help calm the body and mind and facilitate falling asleep. Incorporate these techniques into your nightly routine to let your body know when it's time to relax and get ready for slumber. Exercises that include deep breathing in particular can help induce relaxation and lessen stress and anxiety, which can both impair the quality of sleep.

5. Reduce Alcohol and Caffeine Consumption:

It is well known that alcohol and caffeine can interfere with sleep cycles and reduce the quality of sleep, particularly when they are ingested close to bedtime. To prevent disrupting your sleep, limit the amount of caffeine-containing drinks you consume in the afternoon and evening, such as soda, coffee, and tea. In a similar vein, alcohol can cause fragmented sleep patterns and disturb the regular sleep cycle, even if it may initially make you feel sleepy.

6. Take Part in Regular Exercise:

Sleep length and quality have been demonstrated to increase with regular physical activity. Most days of the week, try to get in at least 30 minutes of moderate-intensity exercise. However, stay away from intense exercise right before bed since it may have an upsetting effect and disrupt your sleep. Including exercises like cycling, yoga, jogging, or walking in your routine can improve your general well-being and quality of sleep.

7. Keep an eye on your diet:

Certain foods and drinks might help or hurt the quality of your sleep. A lot of liquids, hot foods, and big meals should be avoided right before bed because they can make you uncomfortable and interfere with your sleep. Rather, go for light snacks like a small bowl of oats or a banana that are heavy in protein or complex carbs. These can help regulate blood sugar levels and encourage hormones that induce sleep.

8. Control Anxiety and Stress:

Anxiety and stress can have a major negative influence on sleep quality and make it harder to fall asleep and stay asleep all night. Use stress-reduction strategies like journaling, mindfulness meditation, or talking to a therapist or trusted friend about your issues. Before going to bed, practicing relaxation techniques can help ease anxiety and encourage deeper, more restful sleep.

9. Ask for Expert Assistance When Needed:

It could be beneficial to get expert assistance from a healthcare provider or sleep specialist if your sleep issues are not improving even after trying these tactics. They can assess any underlying medical issues or sleep disorders that might be causing your sleep difficulties and suggest the best course of action.

To sum up, improving the quality of your sleep entails forming sound sleeping habits and giving relaxation and stress-reduction strategies a top priority. You may encourage improved sleep hygiene and enhance the quality of your sleep by implementing relaxation techniques, reducing screen time before bed, making your sleep space comfortable, and following a regular sleep routine. Moreover, maintaining a healthy diet, getting regular exercise, and getting aid from a professional when necessary can all help you attain restorative and peaceful sleep.

Examining the Possible Advantages of
Hormone-Regulating Therapies for Better Sleep

Hormone-regulating drugs and treatments, such as hormone replacement therapy (HRT), are frequently used to treat symptoms of hormonal imbalances, including menopause-related symptoms. Although the main goals of these treatments are to control menopausal symptoms such vaginal dryness, hot flashes, and mood swings, they may also have benefits for enhancing sleep quality and resolving sleep problems. Comprehending how hormone-regulating therapies affect sleep can offer valuable perspectives on their possible advantages in attaining rejuvenating and peaceful slumber.

1. Hormonal Level Stabilization:

Menopausal sleep disorders are largely caused by hormonal changes, especially the drop in estrogen levels. Hormone-regulating therapies, including combination estrogen-progestin therapy or estrogen therapy, aim to regulate hormone levels and replicate the premenopausal natural hormonal environment. These therapies can help regulate the body's internal clock and encourage longer and higher-quality sleep by supplying a consistent flow of hormones.

2. Decrease in Night Sweats and Hot Flashes:

During menopause, hot flashes and night sweats are frequent symptoms that can seriously interfere with sleep habits. Hot flashes and night sweats have been demonstrated to be significantly reduced in frequency and severity by hormone-regulating medications, especially estrogen therapy. These treatments can help reduce sleep disruptions and encourage more restful sleep by reducing these symptoms.

3. Mood and Emotional Well-Being Improvement:

Anxiety, irritability, and depression are examples of frequent mood disorders that can affect sleep quality and general well-being during menopause. Hormone-regulating therapies have been demonstrated to enhance menopausal women's mood and emotional health, which may improve their sleep quality. These treatments may indirectly enhance overall sleep satisfaction and sleep quality by addressing symptoms associated with mood.

4. Improving the Architecture of Sleep:

Menopause-related sleep disturbances can upset the regular sleep architecture, resulting in less efficient and fragmented sleep. By encouraging deeper and more restorative sleep stages, such as rapid eye movement (REM) and slow-wave sleep, hormone-regulating therapies may aid in the restoration of regular sleep patterns. These therapies can improve the overall quality of sleep and induce feelings of renewal and refreshment when you wake up by improving the architecture of sleep.

5. Decrease in Stress and Anxiety:

Menopause-related hormonal imbalances can aggravate worry and stress, which in turn can worsen sleep problems. Hormone-regulating therapies can help lessen anxiety and stress by balancing hormone levels and treating symptoms linked to mood. This can lead to a calmer, more relaxed state that is better for sleep. These therapies can improve overall well-being and sleep quality by reducing psychological distress.

6. Achievable Gains in Cognitive Ability:

Menopause-related sleep disruptions can hurt cognitive function, including memory, focus, and decision-making. Hormone-regulating medications may enhance cognitive performance by encouraging longer and higher-quality sleep. These therapies may improve cognitive health and performance by promoting better sleep, which is necessary for cognitive functions like memory consolidation and information processing.

7. Personalized Therapy Choices:

Hormone-regulating medications allow for customized treatment plans based on the requirements and preferences of the patient. Medical professionals can collaborate closely with patients to identify the best hormone therapy plan based on lifestyle considerations, medical history, menopausal symptoms, and age. Patients can optimize the potential advantages of hormone-regulating therapies for better sleep and general well-being by personalizing their treatment options.

In summary, hormone-regulating therapies may be beneficial for enhancing the quality of sleep and treating menopausal-related sleep disorders. These treatments can help improve sleep outcomes and overall sleep satisfaction by stabilizing hormone levels, lowering hot flashes and night sweats, elevating sleep architecture, lowering anxiety and stress, and possibly even improving cognitive function. To choose the best course of action for a patient's needs, it's crucial to consider the possible advantages of hormone therapy against its dangers and adverse effects. You should also consult with your healthcare professional frequently.

Enhancing Mental Well-Being via Mindfulness Exercises

The importance of mental well-being in preserving general health and well-being has grown in the fast-paced world of today. Cultivating mindfulness practices has become a potent technique for promoting mental wellness and enhancing resilience against life's challenges in the face of everyday stressors. We can develop a better sense of awareness, emotional balance, and inner calm by introducing mindfulness into our daily lives. This can promote a good attitude toward life and enhance mental health in general.

1. Acknowledging Mindfulness:

The deliberate attention to the current moment without bias or attachment is known as mindfulness. It entails opening up and becoming curiously aware of our ideas, feelings, physical sensations, and the outside world. Although mindfulness has its roots in antiquated contemplative traditions like Buddhism, it has become more popular as a secular practice with many advantages for mental health in the present era.

2. Mental Wellness Benefits of Mindfulness:

There are several advantages of mindfulness practices for mental health, such as:

- Stress Reduction: By triggering the body's relaxation response, mindfulness practices like body scans and mindful breathing help lower stress chemicals like cortisol and foster a peaceful, relaxed state of mind.
- Emotional Regulation: Mindfulness training helps us become more observant of our thoughts and feelings, which improves our ability to handle difficult situations and control our emotions.
Regular mindfulness practice fosters a greater sense of acceptance, adaptability, and self-compassion in the face of hardship, which increases resilience.
- Increased Focus and Concentration: Mindfulness practices, including mindful

meditation, improve focus and concentration, which boosts mental clarity and productivity.

- Improved Emotional Well-Being: Mindfulness can lessen the signs of anxiety, depression, and other mood disorders while also encouraging happy feelings like joy, kindness, and appreciation.

- Better Sleep Quality: Research has demonstrated that mindfulness-based therapies can enhance the quality of sleep by lowering anxiety, rumination, and pre-sleep arousal. This results in more restful and revitalizing sleep.

- Greater Self-awareness: Mindfulness exercises help us better grasp who we are, what we stand for, and what our deepest desires are. This promotes personal development and increased self-awareness.

3. Including Mindfulness in Everyday Activities:

There is no reason why incorporating mindfulness into our everyday routines has to be difficult or time-consuming. By integrating simple techniques like mindful breathing, mindful eating, or mindful walking into daily routines, we can develop increased awareness and presence all day long. Furthermore, spending a few minutes a day practicing formal mindfulness meditation might offer a chance for more in-depth reflection and relaxation.

4. Interventions Based on Mindfulness:

Mindfulness-Based Stress Reduction (MBSR) and Mindfulness-Based Cognitive Therapy (MBCT) are two examples of mindfulness-based therapies that provide systematic programs for developing mindfulness abilities and advancing mental health. These research-backed therapies combine cognitive-behavioral methods with mindfulness practices to treat a range of mental health issues, including chronic pain, stress, anxiety, and depression.

5. Developing an Intentional Way of Living:

Developing a mindful lifestyle goes beyond formal mindfulness exercises and entails integrating mindfulness into every facet of day-to-day living. This is being totally present in our relationships and experiences, cultivating love, compassion, and thankfulness toward oneself and others, and taking on obstacles with an open mind and lack of judgment. We can develop higher mental wellness and lead more purposeful lives by adopting mindfulness as a way of life.

6. Looking for Expert Advice:

Although mindfulness exercises can help to promote mental wellness, it's important to understand that not everyone can benefit from them and that some people may need further help from mental health specialists. Don't be afraid to seek help from a licensed therapist or counselor if you're having serious problems with your mental health. They can offer you individualized assistance and treatment alternatives that are catered to your requirements.

In summary, developing mental well-being through mindfulness practices provides a comprehensive strategy for developing increased awareness, emotional balance, and resilience in the face of adversity. We can cultivate a greater sense of inner peace, joy, and fulfillment by adopting mindfulness as a way of life and implementing it into our everyday routines. This will enhance our mental and physical health in general.

Taking Up Mindful Activities: Fostering Presence, Awareness, and Well-Being

Adopting mindful practices offers a road to increased awareness, presence, and general well-being in a world full of demands and distractions. Being mindful is consciously focusing on the here and now with acceptance, curiosity, and openness—without passing judgment or being attached to ideas or feelings. We can develop a closer relationship with ourselves and the environment around us by introducing mindful practices into our daily lives. This will boost our clarity, serenity, and ability to bounce back from setbacks.

1. Gaining Knowledge of Mindful Practices:

A vast array of methods and exercises are included in mindful practices to cultivate presence and mindfulness in our daily lives. These techniques incorporate elements of both contemporary modifications and applications in domains like psychology, education, and healthcare, as well as ancient contemplative traditions like yoga and meditation. The fundamental idea is to direct our attention and awareness to the present moment with openness, curiosity, and non-judgment, even though the precise methods may differ.

2. The Advantages of Mindful Activities:

Adopting mindful activities has several wide-ranging advantages that affect our mental, emotional, and physical health in many ways:

- Increased Mental Clarity: Engaging in mindful techniques can help us focus and feel more mentally clear as we go about our everyday lives by calming our minds and reducing mental noise.
- Less Stress and Anxiety: Mindfulness practices encourage relaxation and stress reduction, which lessens tension and anxiety symptoms.
- Improved Emotional Regulation: Mindful techniques help us respond to difficult situations with more emotional balance and composure by raising our awareness of our thoughts and feelings.
- Enhanced Self-awareness: Mindfulness promotes self-analysis and introspection, which results in a better comprehension of our goals, values, and identities.
- Greater Resilience: Consistent mindfulness practice makes us more resilient to life's obstacles by fortifying our capacity to overcome hardship and recover from setbacks.

- Better Relationships: Mindful communication helps us engage with people with empathy, compassion, and understanding, which results in more satisfying and meaningful relationships.
- Improved Physical Health: Research has linked mindfulness to a host of advantages for physical health, such as lowered blood pressure, strengthening immunity, and better sleep.

3. Including Mindfulness in Everyday Activities:

Developing mindful habits doesn't need a large time investment or specialized tools. We may easily incorporate simple practices like mindful walking, mindful eating, and mindful breathing into our regular routines. The secret is to tackle these tasks with focus and intention, using all of our senses and staying mindful of the here and now.

4. Regular Mindfulness Practice:

Formal mindfulness meditation is scheduling specific time for contemplation and silent thought. This can entail guided meditation, in which we adhere to a teacher's instructions or a recorded meditation guide, or seated meditation, in which we concentrate on the breath or other sensations. Formal meditation practice regularly can improve our capacity for mindfulness and give us a sense of serenity and focus in the middle of life's chaos.

5. Consideration in Practice:

Beyond structured meditation, awareness can be applied at any time during our everyday routines. By paying attention to the present moment with awareness and intention, we may incorporate mindfulness into our behaviors, whether we're doing the dishes, walking to work, or chatting with a friend. By engaging in this "mindfulness in action" technique, we may bring more presence and purpose to every area of our lives.

6. Developing an Attitude of Mindfulness:

Developing attentive habits affects not only our actions but also our outlook on life. In our interactions with ourselves and others, we can cultivate attributes like patience, curiosity, and compassion by adopting a mindful mindset. It entails letting go of criticism and judgment to accept each moment for what it is and to embrace it with candor.

7. Getting Past Obstacles and Resistance:

Although implementing mindful practices has many advantages, it's vital to recognize that it won't always be simple. It could take work, self-control, and patience to incorporate mindfulness into our lives, just like any new habit. In addition to external barriers like time limits or doubt from others, we can run across resistance from ourselves. But we can overcome these obstacles and enjoy the benefits of a more mindful way of life if we approach the process with love, persistence, and self-compassion.

8. Looking for Community and Support:

Lastly, it's critical to keep in mind that we don't have to go it alone when pursuing mindfulness. Along the process, accountability, inspiration, and support can be obtained by reaching out to like-minded people through online communities, mindfulness retreats, or meditation groups. We may enhance our practice and increase our sense of belonging by forming relationships with people who share our dedication to mindfulness.

To sum up, implementing mindful practices provides a life-changing route to increased presence, awareness, and well-being. We can fully utilize mindfulness to improve every element of our physical, mental, and emotional well-being by implementing it into our daily routines, developing a mindful mindset, and conquering obstacles with tenacity and self-compassion. May we welcome every moment with openness, love, and curiosity as we proceed on this path of self-awareness and development.

Explain how mindfulness practices may help reduce stress

Stress has become a common and persistent part of many people's everyday lives in today's fast-paced society. Prolonged stress can be harmful to one's physical and emotional well-being, resulting in a variety of symptoms like weariness, anxiety, and even chronic illnesses. Thankfully, mindfulness techniques are a potent remedy for stress, giving people useful skills to control and lessen its negative effects on their well-being. People who practice mindfulness are better able to handle life's obstacles with more composure, resiliency, and inner serenity.

1. Comprehending Stress:

Stress is the body's normal reaction to perceived dangers or difficulties; it sets off a series of physiological and psychological processes that are designed to help us deal with the threat. While short-term stress may be advantageous in some circumstances, long-term or excessive stress can be harmful to our health and well-being. Workplace pressure, money problems, interpersonal disputes, and health issues are just a few of the variables that can cause chronic stress and its host of detrimental effects.

2. Mindfulness's Function in Stress Reduction:

Developing awareness, presence, and acceptance in the present moment is the foundation of mindfulness practices, which provide a comprehensive strategy for stress reduction. Mindfulness assists us in removing ourselves from worrying thoughts about the past or future, which are frequent causes of tension and anxiety, by focusing on the present now. Mindfulness teaches us to watch our thoughts and emotions with inquiry and compassion, allowing them to come and go without being entangled in them, as opposed to getting caught up in a cycle of rumination and concern.

3. Intentional Breathing:

Mindful breathing is among the easiest and most often used mindfulness techniques for stress reduction. We can ground ourselves in the here and now and cultivate a sense of inner peace and relaxation by concentrating on the feelings of the breath as it enters and exits the body. By triggering the body's relaxation response, mindful breathing lowers the release of stress chemicals like cortisol and encourages a state of physiological and psychological balance.

4. Mental Scanning:

The body scan meditation is another useful mindfulness technique for stress reduction. We move methodically through the various body parts in this practice, bringing awareness to any tension or discomfort and allowing it to soften and release with each breath. By practicing the body scan meditation, we can strengthen our bond with our bodies and become more conscious of the outward signs of stress and tension.

5. Conscious Motion:

Gentle physical exercise combined with mindfulness techniques, like yoga, tai chi, or qigong, promotes mental clarity, relaxation, and flexibility. By bringing the breath and movement into harmony, these exercises help us develop a state of relaxation and flow that benefits our bodies and minds. Because mindful movement promotes relaxation, releases muscular tension, and heightens body awareness, it can be very beneficial in lowering stress.

6. Intentional Consumption:

A mindful eating practice entails paying attention to all of the senses involved in the eating process, such as the taste, texture, and aroma of the meal as well as the feelings of fullness and hunger. We may create a more balanced and intuitive eating style and have a deeper appreciation for food by taking our time and enjoying every bite. By encouraging a sense of fullness, satisfaction, and connection to our bodies, mindful eating can help lower stress.

7. MBSR (Mindfulness-Based Stress Reduction)*

Dr. Jon Kabat-Zinn created the structured program known as Mindfulness-Based Stress Reduction (MBSR), which incorporates mindfulness techniques into an all-encompassing strategy for stress management and well-being promotion. MBSR incorporates instruction on stress physiology and coping mechanisms with body awareness exercises, mindfulness meditation, and gentle movement techniques. MBSR has been shown in numerous trials to be beneficial in lowering stress, anxiety, and depression symptoms as well as enhancing general quality of life.

8. Cognizance in Everyday Life:

Beyond structured meditation techniques, mindfulness may be used in all facets of our daily lives, from routine activities like walking or dishwashing to more difficult circumstances like handling difficult emotions or conflicts. A stronger sense of presence, acceptance, and resilience in the face of stressors can be developed by incorporating mindful awareness into our daily actions and interactions.

9. Looking for Expert Advice:

Although mindfulness exercises can be helpful in lowering stress, it's vital to understand that not everyone can benefit from them and that some people might need further help from mental health specialists. Don't be afraid to seek help from a licensed therapist or counselor if you're dealing with severe discomfort or persistent stress. They can offer you individualized assistance and treatment alternatives that are catered to your requirements.

In summary, mindfulness exercises provide a potent and practical strategy for lowering stress and enhancing general well-being. We can improve our emotional balance, inner serenity, and resilience to life's obstacles by practicing awareness, presence, and acceptance in the here and now. Whether we do this through formal meditation practices, mindful movement, or just applying mindful awareness to our everyday activities, integrating mindfulness into our lives can make it easier for us to manage stress and lead more effortless, energetic lives.

Talk about how mental health affects menopausal experience

Mental Health's Effect on Menopausal Experience

A woman's menopause ushers in a new period of hormonal shifts and physical modifications, marking the end of her reproductive years. It is a momentous time in a woman's life. Menopause has a profound effect on mental and emotional health, even though it is a normal aspect of aging. A woman's mental health during this transitional time can be greatly influenced by the interplay of hormonal variations, physical symptoms, and psychosocial variables, which in turn shape her whole menopausal experience.

1. Mood swings and hormonal fluctuations:

The beginning of mood swings and emotional problems during menopause is largely caused by hormonal imbalances, especially the decrease in estrogen levels. The reduction of estrogen during menopause can cause dysregulation of neurotransmitters like dopamine and serotonin, which are implicated in mood regulation. Estrogen is known to have neuroprotective and mood-regulating properties. As a result, throughout the menopausal transition, a lot of women experience mood swings, irritability, anxiety, and even melancholy.

2. Social Significance and Mental Effects:

Menopause-related physical symptoms, like vaginal dryness, hot flashes, night sweats, and sleep problems, can significantly affect a woman's quality of life and mental health. For example, persistent sleep disruptions can aggravate mood disorders and cognitive decline, making it more difficult to feel rested, irritable, and emotionally unstable. Likewise, emotions of low self-worth, discontent, and despair may be exacerbated by ongoing physical discomfort and modifications in body image.

3. Stressors and Psychosocial Factors:

Stressors in life and psychosocial variables can worsen mental health problems during menopause. A variety of stressors that women may encounter in their lives—work, family, relationships, and caregiving duties—can exacerbate feelings of overload, anxiety, and burnout. Furthermore, ageism, stigma, and other unfavorable cultural views surrounding menopause can hurt mental health and lead to negative self-perceptions.

4. Impact on Residing and Operating Conditions:

Menopause-related mental health issues can have a serious negative influence on a woman's general functioning and quality of life. Mood disorders and psychiatric symptoms that are left untreated can affect everyday functioning, productivity at work, interpersonal connections, and general quality of life. Women may experience difficulties adjusting to the demands of daily life, retreat from social interactions, and have trouble maintaining interpersonal relationships.

5. Singular Dissimilarities and Weaknesses:

Menopause is a highly personalized experience, and women differ in how susceptible they are to mental health problems depending on a range of factors including genetics, personal history, lifestyle choices, and social support systems. Women who already suffer from mental health issues, like anxiety or depression, may be more likely to have their menopausal symptoms worsen. In a similar vein, women who have experienced major trauma or stress in their lives may be particularly susceptible to mental health issues during this time of change.

6. Looking for Assistance and Care:

Menopausal mental health concerns necessitate a thorough and integrated strategy that takes into account the biological, psychological, and social underlying causes of symptoms. Women who are experiencing severe distress or functional impairment should contact a qualified healthcare provider, such as a mental health specialist, gynecologist, or primary care physician. To reduce symptoms and enhance general well-being, treatment options may include hormone therapy, psychotherapy, medication, lifestyle changes, and complementary therapies.

7. Caring for Oneself and Coping Mechanisms:

Women can manage their mental health during menopause by practicing self-care and coping mechanisms in addition to seeking professional help. This could entail engaging in stress-reduction practices including deep breathing, mindfulness meditation, and relaxation exercises. Mental resilience and well-being can also be enhanced by frequent physical activity, eating a balanced diet, getting enough sleep, and asking friends and family for social support.

8. Advocacy and Empowerment:

Educating women about menopause and mental health is essential to fostering advocacy, self-awareness, and resilience. Women who are aware of the typical menopausal symptoms and difficulties will be better able to identify when they may want assistance and seek out the right resources and therapies. Reducing obstacles to care and fostering a more understanding and supportive social environment can also be achieved by advocating for increased knowledge and destigmatization of menopause-related mental health disorders.

In conclusion, a woman's menopausal experience is greatly influenced by her mental health. The intricate relationship between menopause and mental health is influenced by a variety of factors, including individual susceptibility, psychosocial variables, physical symptoms, and oscillations in hormone levels. Women may move into menopause with increased resilience, empowerment, and general well-being if mental health concerns are treated with empathy, understanding, and evidence-based interventions.

Examine how therapy can help with emotional support and change management

Analyzing Therapy's Function in Supporting Emotions and Encouraging Change Management

In times of change and transition, therapy, in all of its forms and modalities, is a helpful tool for people looking for emotional support and direction. Therapy provides a secure and private setting for investigation, introspection, and development, whether dealing with mental health concerns, psychological obstacles, or life transitions like job shifts, marital problems, or health issues. Through the development of coping mechanisms, self-awareness, and positive transformation, therapy can equip people to face life's obstacles with increased emotional stability, resilience, and self-efficacy.

1. Validation and Emotional Support:

Offering emotional support and affirmation to those who are going through difficult times, uncertainty, or life changes is one of the main purposes of therapy. Therapists provide a kind and accepting environment in which clients can communicate their ideas, emotions, and worries without worrying about being judged or rejected. Therapists assist clients in feeling seen, heard, and understood by using active listening, empathy, and validation. This builds the safety and trust that are necessary for therapeutic advancement.

2. Inquiry and Self-Revelation:

In therapy, people can thoroughly examine their ideas, values, actions, and beliefs in a controlled and encouraging setting. Clients can learn more about their inner selves and the things that shape their beliefs and behaviors by engaging in introspective tasks, guided reflection, and open communication with their therapist. Greater self-awareness, self-acceptance, and clarity regarding one's objectives, ambitions, and aspirations are fostered by this process of self-discovery.

3. Building Resilience and Coping Skills:

Therapy gives people useful coping mechanisms and resilience-boosting techniques to help them deal with life's obstacles more skillfully. To help their clients regulate their emotions, deal with stress, and find constructive solutions to problems, therapists teach them evidence-based approaches like mindfulness exercises, cognitive-behavioral coping skills, stress management strategies, and communication skills. Through recognizing and questioning harmful thought patterns, controlling emotions, and using assertive communication, clients strengthen their emotional fortitude and acquire flexible coping mechanisms.

4. Goal-setting and Change Management:

Through goal-setting, action planning, and the use of techniques for constructive transformation, therapy helps people manage transition and change. Therapists work with clients to discover their values, abilities, and resources while they navigate job changes, relationship adjustments, or health issues. Together, they create a plan for reaching the goals that the clients have set for themselves. Therapy gives individuals the tools they need to take proactive measures toward their own personal development and transformation through goal-setting, problem-solving, and accountability.

5. Managing Trauma and Bereavement:

Therapy offers a secure and encouraging environment for people to grieve loss, unresolved grief, and traumatic events. To assist clients in integrating difficult feelings, healing from emotional scars, and exploring and making meaning of their experiences, therapists employ evidence-based techniques such as expressive arts therapy, bereavement counseling, and trauma-focused therapy. Therapists help clients heal and regain their sense of agency and resilience by providing them with sympathetic support and validation.

6. Creating Resources and Support Networks:

To improve their emotional health and resilience, therapy can assist people in creating support systems and gaining access to resources. Depending on the requirements and desires of their clients, therapists may recommend them to specialized programs, support groups, or other community resources. To build stronger, more supportive social networks, therapists also collaborate with their clients to help them set boundaries, practice assertive communication, and improve their interpersonal connections.

7. Encouraging Self-Care and Self-Compassion:

Self-care and self-compassion are encouraged in therapy as vital elements of emotional health and resiliency. Through challenging self-critical ideas and fostering self-acceptance and self-kindness, therapists assist clients in developing a compassionate and nurturing relationship with themselves. By engaging in self-care activities like mindfulness training, relaxation techniques, and hobbies, clients refuel their emotional reserves and learn to prioritize their well-being, which improves their ability to handle stress and hardship.

8. Eongated Development and Sustaining:

Beyond crisis response or temporary symptom relief, therapy provides an opportunity for sustained emotional well-being and growth. Many people use therapy as a tool for self-improvement, self-discovery, and maintaining their mental health as part of their regular self-care routine. Therapy aids individuals in maintaining positive changes and navigating life's ups and downs with more resilience and self-awareness through frequent check-ins, goal reassessment, and continual skill-building.

To sum up, therapy is essential for helping people deal with the ups and downs of life by offering them emotional support and helping them manage change. Therapy enables people to develop self-awareness, coping mechanisms, and the ability to go through change with more resilience and well-being by providing a secure and private setting for investigation, validation, and development. Therapy is a useful tool for people who are dedicated to their emotional well-being and fulfillment, whether they are looking for assistance

with particular problems or want to engage in
long-term personal development.

Chapter 7

An explanation of hormone replacement therapy (HRT)

A Synopsis of Hormone Replacement Treatment (HRT)

A typical medical treatment for symptoms related to hormonal imbalances, especially during menopause or in cases of hormonal shortage, is hormone replacement therapy (HRT). Hormone replacement therapy (HRT) is a technique used to augment the body's natural hormone levels and treat symptoms like mood swings, vaginal dryness, hot flashes, and night sweats. The hormones administered are usually estrogen, progesterone, or a mix of both. HRT is still a popular and useful therapy option for treating menopausal symptoms and enhancing the quality of life for many, despite current controversy and debate surrounding its possible hazards and benefits.

1. Hormone Replacement Therapy Types:

There are several ways that hormone replacement therapy can be used, such as:

- Estrogen Therapy: Women who have had a hysterectomy (the surgical removal of the uterus) are administered estrogen alone as part of estrogen therapy. It is possible to deliver estrogen therapy orally, transdermally (using gels or patches), or vaginally (with creams, pills, or rings).
- Estrogen-Progestin Therapy: Also referred to as combined hormone therapy, estrogen-progestin therapy is the process of giving progesterone and estrogen to women who have not had a hysterectomy. To guard against the possible negative effects of estrogen alone on the endometrium, and the lining of the uterus, progestin is administered. There are several ways to deliver this combination therapy: as oral tablets, patches, lotions, or vaginal preparations.
- Bioidentical Hormone Therapy: In this type of therapy, hormones that are structurally identical to those the body produces naturally are used. Usually made from plant sources, these hormones are blended to correspond with each person's hormone levels. A prescription for bioidentical hormone therapy may be written for pills, lotions, gels, or subcutaneously inserted pellets.

2. Hormone Replacement Therapy Indications

The main indication for hormone replacement therapy is the treatment of menopausal symptoms, such as mood swings, vaginal dryness, hot flashes, and night sweats. HRT may also be recommended to treat or prevent osteoporosis, a condition in which the bones thin, and lower the risk of fractures in postmenopausal women. In some circumstances, people with disorders like hypogonadism or premature ovarian failure may also take HRT to treat their hormonal deficiencies.

3. Action Mechanism:

To treat symptoms related to hormone imbalances, hormone replacement therapy supplements the body's natural hormone levels. By restoring the body's diminishing estrogen levels throughout menopause, estrogen therapy can lessen symptoms like mood swings, hot flashes, and dry vaginas. To shield the endometrium from the possible negative effects of estrogen alone, such as endometrial hyperplasia (thickening of the uterine lining), progestin is added to estrogen therapy.

4. Potential Dangers and Advantages:

Hormone replacement therapy (HRT) has been linked to possible hazards as well as advantages. Depending on a person's age, medical history, and preferences, the decision to begin HRT should be taken individually. HRT has been demonstrated to successfully lessen the symptoms of menopause and lower the chance of fractures caused by osteoporosis, but it may also come with some hazards, such as an increased risk of breast cancer, blood clots, stroke, and cardiovascular events. Before beginning treatment, the advantages and disadvantages of HRT should be thoroughly considered and addressed with a healthcare professional.

5. Observation and Investigation:

Patients receiving hormone replacement therapy should have routine check-ups with their physician to determine the effectiveness of the medication, keep an eye out for any side effects, and modify the plan of care as necessary. Periodic physical exams, blood tests to measure hormone levels and metabolic parameters, and conversations regarding symptoms and treatment objectives are some examples of monitoring. Physicians may also suggest routine bone density tests, pelvic examinations, and mammograms to check for

possible side effects of hormone replacement
therapy.

6. Thoughts and Possible Solutions:

Hormone replacement therapy may not be
appropriate for all patients; those with certain
medical issues or risk factors should consider other
treatments. Herbal remedies like black cohosh and
soy isoflavones, dietary supplements like vitamin D
and calcium, prescription drugs like selective
serotonin reuptake inhibitors for mood disorders,
and lifestyle changes like diet and exercise are
examples of non-hormonal therapies for managing
menopausal symptoms. Those who are thinking
about hormone replacement treatment should
speak with a healthcare professional about their
alternatives and make an educated choice based on
their requirements and preferences.

To sum up, hormone replacement therapy is a
medical intervention that is frequently
recommended to address symptoms related to
hormonal imbalances, especially during
menopause. While many people find that HRT
improves their quality of life and helps control
menopausal symptoms, it's vital to consider the
potential hazards and benefits and talk with a

healthcare specialist about your alternatives.
Healthcare professionals can collaborate with
patients to create a customized treatment plan that
maximizes symptom alleviation and reduces risks
by carefully taking into account each person's needs
and preferences.

debunking rumors about hormone replacement
therapy (HRT)

Over the years, hormone replacement therapy
(HRT) has generated a great deal of discussion and
controversy due to several myths and
misconceptions regarding its efficacy, safety, and
possible hazards. Even though hormone
replacement therapy (HRT) is a popular treatment
for menopausal symptoms and hormonal
imbalances, it's critical to distinguish fact from
myth to utilize HRT wisely. By busting myths
around HRT, we may increase knowledge of its
advantages and disadvantages and provide people
the power to make informed decisions about their
health.

1. Myth: Hormone replacement treatment should never be used and is always dangerous.

Fact: Hormone replacement therapy is a safe and useful therapeutic choice for many women who are suffering from menopausal symptoms or hormonal imbalances, while it may not be appropriate for everyone. Individual considerations should be given to HRT decisions, including age, medical history, and personal preferences. The advantages of hormone replacement therapy (HRT) in reducing symptoms and enhancing quality of life may exceed the possible hazards for certain women.

2. Myth: Cancer is caused by hormone replacement therapy.

Fact: There have been worries that hormone replacement therapy (HRT) could raise the risk of several malignancies, especially breast cancer. Long-term use of combination estrogen-progestin therapy has been linked in certain studies to a slight increase in breast cancer risk; however, the absolute risk is modest, especially in younger women and those who have never had breast cancer before. Additionally, stopping HRT lowers the risk of breast cancer. When thinking about HRT, it's crucial to go over specific risk concerns and advantages with a healthcare professional.

3. Myth: Weight gain is a result of hormone replacement therapy.

Fact: There isn't enough proof to conclude that hormone replacement therapy (HRT) causes weight gain, even though some women may gain weight or have changes in their body composition after menopause. In fact, by lowering stress and enhancing sleep quality, hormone replacement therapy (HRT) may help manage symptoms like hot flashes and night sweats, which can have an indirect effect on weight control. Individual reactions to HRT may differ, just like with any drug, thus weight fluctuations should be tracked and discussed with a healthcare professional.

4. Myth: Women with severe menopausal symptoms are the only ones who should receive hormone replacement therapy.

Fact: Women who experience mild to severe menopausal symptoms might be offered hormone replacement treatment. Some women may benefit from the symptom relief that hormone replacement therapy (HRT) offers, while others may prefer to manage their symptoms through lifestyle changes or other therapies. Regardless of the severity of their symptoms, women who have a higher risk of osteoporosis or fractures may also benefit from HRT. Individual symptoms, preferences, and risk factors should be taken into consideration while deciding whether to start HRT.

5. Myth: The only way to address menopausal symptoms is with hormone replacement therapy.

Fact: There are other options available for treating menopausal symptoms than hormone replacement therapy, which is a standard treatment. Hot flashes, nocturnal sweats, and vaginal dryness are just a few of the symptoms that can be lessened with a variety of non-hormonal treatments and lifestyle changes. These could include prescription drugs such as selective serotonin reuptake inhibitors (SSRIs), acupuncture, herbal supplements, cognitive-behavioral therapy, and dietary adjustments. Menopausal symptoms sufferers ought to talk over their alternatives with a medical professional to find the best course of action for their circumstances.

6. Myth: Women undergoing natural menopause
are the only ones eligible for hormone replacement
therapy.

Fact: Women who have menopausal symptoms as
a result of premature ovarian insufficiency, surgical
menopause (coming from ovaries being removed),
or natural menopause may be offered hormone
replacement therapy. Regardless of the underlying
cause, hormone replacement therapy (HRT) can
help women experiencing hormonal shortages
reduce symptoms and enhance their quality of life.
However, the choice to start HRT should consider
the patient's medical history, risk factors, and
desired course of treatment.

7. Myth: There are always cardiovascular hazards
linked with hormone replacement therapy.

Fact: The evidence is mixed and contradictory,
although certain studies have expressed concerns
about the cardiovascular risks linked with hormone
replacement treatment, especially in older women
or those who already have cardiovascular disease.
Age, the time of beginning, the length of usage, and
underlying cardiovascular risk factors are some of
the variables that may affect the risk-benefit profile
of hormone replacement therapy. The

cardiovascular advantages of hormone replacement therapy (HRT), including better lipid profiles and a lower risk of osteoporotic fractures, may exceed the possible dangers for certain women. When thinking about HRT, it's crucial to go over the advantages and risks of cardiovascular disease with a healthcare professional.

To sum up, debunking misconceptions regarding hormone replacement therapy is crucial to advancing knowledge of its application in the treatment of menopausal symptoms and hormonal dysregulation. When used properly, hormone replacement therapy (HRT) can be a safe and successful treatment choice for many women, while it may not be appropriate for everyone and carries certain hazards. Menopausal symptom sufferers can live better lives and achieve optimal outcomes if we provide them with correct information and the empowerment to make health-related decisions.

Misunderstandings about HRT and its advantages and disadvantages.

Explicating Frequently Held Myths About Hormone Replacement Therapy (HRT) and Its Benefits and Drawbacks

The safety, effectiveness, and possible hazards of hormone replacement therapy (HRT) have long been the subject of debate and controversy. While hormone replacement therapy (HRT) can be an effective treatment for menopausal symptoms and hormonal imbalances, it's important to dispel myths and give people accurate information so they can make decisions about their health. We may encourage a better knowledge of this therapeutic strategy and its role in women's health by discussing the benefits and drawbacks of hormone replacement therapy (HRT) and clearing up common misconceptions.

1. Misunderstanding: HRT is never safe and ought to be stayed away from.

To be clear, hormone replacement therapy (HRT) can be a safe and effective therapeutic choice for many women experiencing menopausal symptoms or hormonal shortages, but it may not be appropriate for everyone and carries some risks. A person's age, medical history, and preferences should all be taken into consideration when deciding whether to start HRT. HRT may be more advantageous for some women than harmful in terms of symptom relief and quality of life enhancement.

2. Misunderstanding: Cancer is caused by HRT.

To be clear, there have been worries that hormone replacement therapy (HRT) could raise the risk of some malignancies, especially breast cancer. Long-term use of combination estrogen-progestin therapy has been linked in certain studies to a slight increase in breast cancer risk; however, the absolute risk is modest, especially in younger women and those who have never had breast cancer before. Additionally, stopping HRT lowers the risk of breast cancer. When thinking about HRT, it's crucial to go over specific risk concerns and advantages with a healthcare professional.

3. Hormone replacement therapy leads to weight gain.

Clarification: There is no conclusive evidence to support the theory that hormone replacement therapy (HRT) causes weight gain, even though some women may gain weight or see changes in their body composition after menopause. In fact, by lowering stress and enhancing sleep quality, hormone replacement therapy (HRT) may help manage symptoms like hot flashes and night sweats, which can have an indirect effect on weight control. Individual reactions to HRT may differ, just like with any drug, thus weight fluctuations should be tracked and discussed with a healthcare professional.

4. Misconception: The only way to treat menopausal symptoms is with hormone replacement therapy.

To be clear, hormone replacement therapy (HRT) is not the only treatment for menopausal symptoms. Hot flashes, nocturnal sweats, and vaginal dryness are just a few of the symptoms that can be lessened with a variety of non-hormonal treatments and lifestyle changes. These could include prescription drugs such as selective serotonin reuptake inhibitors (SSRIs), acupuncture, herbal supplements, cognitive-behavioral therapy, and dietary adjustments. Menopausal symptoms sufferers ought to talk over their alternatives with a medical professional to find the best course of action for their circumstances.

5. There is always a danger of cardiovascular disease with hormone replacement therapy.

To be clear, there is inconsistent and complicated information supporting the claims made by certain studies regarding the cardiovascular risks linked to hormone replacement therapy (HRT), especially for older women or those who already have cardiovascular disease. Age, the time of beginning, the length of usage, and underlying cardiovascular risk factors are some of the variables that may affect the risk-benefit profile of hormone replacement therapy. The cardiovascular advantages of hormone replacement therapy (HRT), including better lipid profiles and a lower risk of osteoporotic fractures, may exceed the possible dangers for certain women. When thinking about HRT, it's crucial to go over the advantages and risks of cardiovascular disease with a healthcare professional.

HRT benefits include: - Reduction of menopausal symptoms, including mood swings, vaginal dryness, hot flashes, and night sweats.
Osteoporosis therapy and prevention, as well as lower risk of fracture.
- An increase in the standard of living and general health for a large number of women who suffer from hormone abnormalities.

HRT drawbacks include: a raised risk of blood clots, stroke, cardiovascular events, and breast cancer, among other illnesses.

- Possible adverse effects include headache, nausea, bloating, and breast tenderness.
Regular monitoring and follow-up are required to evaluate the effectiveness of treatment, keep an eye out for side effects, and modify it as necessary.

Finally, even though hormone replacement therapy can be an effective treatment for menopausal symptoms and hormonal imbalances, it's critical to clear up common misconceptions and give factual information about the benefits and drawbacks of the procedure. Women can decide if HRT is the best option for them by talking with a healthcare professional about their risk factors, treatment objectives, and preferences. In the end, deciding to start HRT should be based on carefully weighing the advantages and disadvantages of the procedure as well as the available alternatives.

Examine how hormone treatment may be used to treat menopausal symptoms.

Analyzing the Hormone Treatment Option for Menopausal Symptom Management

Due to hormonal changes, menopause—the natural end of a woman's reproductive years—is frequently accompanied by a variety of uncomfortable symptoms. Menopausal hormone therapy (MHT), also referred to as hormone replacement therapy (HRT), is a popular method for treating menopausal symptoms and enhancing quality of life. Hormone therapy is an effective way to address a range of menopausal symptoms, from mood swings and vaginal dryness to hot flashes and night sweats. Hormone therapy works by replenishing diminishing hormone levels. Let's look at how these typical menopausal symptoms might be treated with hormone therapy:

1. Night sweats and hot flashes:

Among menopausal women's most common and bothersome symptoms are hot flashes and nocturnal sweats. These unexpected, strong heat waves can cause flushing, sweating, and discomfort. They can also cause sleep disturbances and interfere with daily tasks. Hot flashes and night sweats can be significantly reduced in frequency and intensity with hormone therapy, especially estrogen therapy. Hormone therapy lowers the frequency and severity of vasomotor symptoms by stabilizing the body's internal thermostat by restoring the body's diminishing estrogen levels.

2. Atrophy and Dryness in the Vagina:

Thinning, inflamed, and dry vaginal tissues are common signs of estrogen shortage after menopause, which can lead to vaginal dryness and atrophy. Vaginal itching, pain during sexual activity, and a higher risk of urinary tract infections can result from these symptoms. To relieve the symptoms of vaginal dryness and discomfort, estrogen therapy can be applied locally using vaginal creams, pills, or rings. These methods can successfully restore vaginal moisture, suppleness, and lubrication.

3. Disturbances in Sleep:

Menopausal women commonly suffer sleep disorders, such as insomnia, fragmented sleep, and nocturnal awakenings, which are typically linked to mood swings, night sweats, and hormonal changes. By lowering nocturnal hot flashes and night sweats, encouraging relaxation, and regulating mood, hormone therapy may help increase the quantity and quality of sleep. Hormone therapy alleviates uncomfortable menopausal symptoms, which can improve general well-being and the quality of sleep.

4. Emotional Shifts and Anger Management:

Menopausal women frequently experience mood swings, anger, and emotional instability, which are frequently linked to hormonal changes, sleep issues, and pressures in life. Hormone therapy, especially estrogen therapy, has been demonstrated to stabilize hormone levels, improve neurotransmitter function, and lessen irritability and mood disorders. Hormone therapy can assist women manage the emotional difficulties of menopause by encouraging emotional stability and resilience.

5. Orthoporosis Prevention and Bone Health:

Menopause-related declines in estrogen levels can hasten bone loss and raise the risk of osteoporosis, a disorder marked by porous, brittle bones and a heightened vulnerability to fractures. In women going through menopause, hormone therapy—especially estrogen-progestin therapy—can help maintain bone density, lower the incidence of osteoporotic fractures, and improve skeletal health. Hormone therapy helps preserve bone strength and integrity by promoting bone formation and blocking bone resorption, which lowers the risk of fractures and consequences from osteoporosis.

6. Memory and Cognitive Function:

Some women going through menopause report experiencing memory problems and cognitive abnormalities, although it's still unclear how much menopause causes cognitive loss. It has been proposed that hormone therapy, especially estrogen therapy, may increase verbal memory, attention span, and executive function, among other cognitive functions. To clarify the connection between hormone therapy and cognitive results, more study is necessary as the information about the effects of hormone treatment on menopausal women's cognitive performance is conflicting.

In summary, hormone therapy is a useful and successful strategy for controlling menopausal symptoms and enhancing menopausal women's quality of life. Hormone therapy can relieve several symptoms, such as mood swings, sleep difficulties, vaginal dryness, hot flashes, and night sweats, by replenishing diminishing hormone levels. To choose the best course of action for controlling menopausal symptoms based on personal needs, preferences, and medical history, it's crucial to consider the possible advantages and disadvantages of hormone therapy and talk with a healthcare professional about each treatment choice.

Hormone Harmony: Examine the many hormone treatments that are available and talk about how individualized hormone control may enhance general wellbeing.

Hormone Harmony: Examining the Variety of Hormone Therapies and the Advantages of Tailored Hormone Management for Overall Health

The human body's complex hormonal dance is essential for controlling a range of physiological functions, including mood, sleep, and reproduction as well as metabolism. This delicate equilibrium can be upset by hormone imbalances, which are frequently linked to diseases like menopause, hormonal disorders, or aging. This can result in a wide range of symptoms and health issues. Thankfully, developments in medicine have produced a wide range of hormone therapies intended to correct hormonal imbalances and enhance general health. Healthcare professionals can improve overall welfare and maximize treatment success by customizing hormone therapy to each patient's requirements and preferences.

1. Hormone Treatment Types:

A wide range of therapeutic approaches are included in hormone therapies, all of which have as their goal adjusting hormone levels to treat particular medical conditions or reduce symptoms brought on by hormonal imbalances. The following are a few typical hormone treatment types:

- Hormone Replacement Therapy (HRT): HRT is the process of supplementing low hormone levels with hormones like progesterone, estrogen, or testosterone to relieve symptoms related to hypogonadism, menopause, and other hormonal deficiencies.

Bioidentical Hormone Therapy: This treatment method makes use of hormones that have the same structural makeup as the body's hormones. These plant-based hormones can be prescribed as creams, gels, pills, or pellets. They are customized to meet each patient's unique hormone levels.

- Thyroid Hormone Replacement: To replace low thyroid hormone levels in people with hypothyroidism or thyroid disorders, synthetic thyroid hormones, such as levothyroxine or liothyronine, are administered.

- Growth Hormone Therapy: To treat growth hormone shortages or conditions like short stature or growth hormone deficiency linked to aging or specific medical conditions, recombinant human growth hormone (GH) is administered.

- Insulin Therapy: Exogenous insulin injections or insulin analogs are used in conjunction with the body's natural insulin production to replace or enhance the body's insulin production to control blood sugar levels and avert complications related to diabetes.

2. Personalized Hormone Regulation and Health:

The idea of tailored treatment, which acknowledges that hormone requirements and responses differ greatly amongst people depending on variables including age, sex, heredity, lifestyle, and medical history, is one of the fundamental tenets of hormone therapy. Healthcare professionals can improve overall well-being, decrease side effects, and maximize treatment outcomes by customizing hormone therapy to each patient's needs and preferences. Individualized hormone management may improve overall health in several ways, including:

- Symptom Relief: Personalized hormone therapy enables medical professionals to focus on the unique symptoms or health issues that each patient faces, such as hot flashes, mood swings, exhaustion, or sexual dysfunction. Through specialized hormone therapy, people can significantly alleviate these symptoms and improve their general quality of life.

- Hormonal Balance: An imbalance in hormones can cause several physiological problems and be a contributing factor in several health problems, such as mood disorders, reproductive disorders, and metabolic disorders. By bringing hormone levels back into optimal ranges, personalized hormone control seeks to promote general health and wellness by reestablishing hormonal balance.

- Personalized Approach: To create a customized treatment plan that meets each patient's specific needs and addresses their individual issues, personalized hormone therapy considers each patient's unique medical history, lifestyle circumstances, preferences, and treatment goals. With this individualized approach, patients are guaranteed to receive the most suitable and efficient hormone therapy based on their unique situation.

- Preventive Health Benefits: By lowering the risk of illnesses like osteoporosis, cardiovascular disease, and cognitive decline that are linked to hormonal imbalances, hormone therapy can also have a preventive effect on health. Individualized hormone control can help avoid or delay the onset of age-related health disorders and promote healthy aging by optimizing hormone levels and improving general health and vigor.

3. Navigating Options for Hormone Treatment:

Hormone therapy has many advantages for improving overall health, but treatment choices must be carefully thought through and discussed with a licensed healthcare professional. It is important for patients to actively participate in conversations regarding their treatment options, including any possible advantages, disadvantages, and substitutes for hormone therapy. To find the best hormone treatment for each patient, medical professionals should perform comprehensive assessments that include risk assessments, physical exams, lab testing, and medical histories.

In addition, continuous monitoring and follow-up are crucial to guarantee the effectiveness and safety of hormone therapy and to modify the treatment plan as needed in response to the patient's changing demands. People can confidently explore hormone treatment options and maximize their overall well-being by working with an informed and competent healthcare professional and actively participating in their treatment decisions.

To sum up, hormone therapy provides a wide range of therapeutic alternatives for resolving hormonal imbalances and enhancing overall health. Healthcare practitioners can maximize treatment success, reduce side effects, and improve patients' overall quality of life by customizing hormone therapy to each patient's needs and preferences. An individual's journey toward optimal health and vitality can be supported by achieving hormonal balance, symptom relief, and preventive health advantages through a tailored approach to hormone control.

Emphasizing the Value of Making Informed Decisions and Performing Regular Checks in Hormone Therapy

When it comes to hormone therapy, making educated decisions and checking frequently is essential to guaranteeing the treatment's safety, effectiveness, and overall success. Hormone therapy, including thyroid hormone replacement, hormone replacement therapy (HRT) for menopause, and other forms of hormone modulation, has advantages and disadvantages that need to be carefully examined and tracked over time. By highlighting the importance of patients and healthcare providers being watchful and proactive, we can avoid potential issues related to hormone therapy and encourage optimal outcomes.

1. Educated Choice-Making:

The first step in making an informed decision is comprehending the goals, advantages, and possible drawbacks of hormone therapy. When thinking about hormone therapy, patients should have in-depth conversations with their medical professionals to assess the possible advantages of the procedure against any hazards. Patients must actively participate in the decision-making process and have a thorough grasp of all available treatment alternatives, including alternative therapies.

Healthcare professionals are essential in helping patients make educated decisions about hormone therapy by giving correct information, responding to inquiries, and resolving concerns. In order to

provide patients the power to make decisions that
are in line with their preferences and treatment
objectives, they should inform them about the
indications for treatment, possible side effects, and
long-term implications of hormone therapy.

2. Continuous Surveillance and Monitoring:

Regular monitoring and follow-up appointments
are crucial for evaluating the effectiveness of
treatment, keeping an eye out for any adverse
effects, and modifying the treatment plan as
needed. Healthcare professionals should keep a
careful eye on patients receiving hormone therapy
to make sure that hormone levels stay within
therapeutic ranges and that any side effects are
quickly detected and treated.

Regular physical exams, lab work to measure
hormone levels and metabolic markers, and
conversations regarding the status of treatment,
any changes in symptoms, and the patient's overall
health are all possible components of monitoring.
Clear guidelines for monitoring patients receiving
hormone therapy should be established by
healthcare professionals, who should also inform
patients of the need to keep follow-up

appointments and report any worrisome symptoms or changes in their health.

3. Personalized Care Plans:

Customized treatment strategies are crucial for maximizing the safety and effectiveness of hormone therapy as each patient is unique. Treatment plans should be customized for each patient by medical professionals based on their unique needs, taking into consideration things like age, medical history, hormone levels, treatment objectives, and preferences. Healthcare professionals can optimize the advantages of hormone therapy and reduce the possibility of side effects by creating personalized treatment regimens for each patient.

Personalized treatment plans may include determining the best hormone formulation, dosage, and delivery method depending on the unique needs of each patient and the goals of the treatment. Treatment regimens should also include routine monitoring and modifications as necessary to guarantee that patients continue to achieve the best possible results during therapy and that hormone levels stay within target ranges.

4. Collaborative Decision-Making and Empowered
Patients:

Effective hormone therapy requires patient
empowerment and shared decision-making.
Patients ought to be actively involved in the course
of their care, given the chance to express their
preferences, pose inquiries, and weigh in on choices
pertaining to their care. In order to provide patients
the confidence to actively manage their own health
and wellness, healthcare practitioners should
cultivate an environment of open communication,
mutual respect, and teamwork.

Healthcare practitioners can improve treatment
adherence, satisfaction, and outcomes by
incorporating patients in shared decision-making
processes. Patients are more likely to follow
treatment recommendations, express their
concerns honestly, and take an active role in their
healthcare journey if they feel empowered,
informed, and supported.

To guarantee safe, effective, and customized
treatment in hormone therapy, emphasize the need
to make educated decisions and do periodic
checkups. Together, patients and healthcare
professionals must take an active role in managing

their treatment, committing to proactive management of hormone therapy, frequent monitoring, and well-informed decision-making. Hormone therapy patients can have better outcomes and a higher quality of life if we prioritize patient empowerment, education, and communication.

Establishing a Network of Support: Enhancing Wellbeing Through Community and Connection

In navigating life's challenges, having a strong network of support can make all the difference in promoting resilience, fostering emotional well-being, and enhancing overall quality of life. This is particularly true when it comes to managing health-related issues, including those associated with hormone therapy, where emotional, practical, and informational support can play a crucial role in the treatment journey. By establishing a network of support, individuals undergoing hormone therapy can access the resources, encouragement, and understanding they need to navigate the complexities of treatment and thrive.

1. Types of Support Networks:

Support networks can take various forms, encompassing different types of relationships, communities, and resources. Some common types of support networks include:

- Family and Friends: Family members, friends, and loved ones can provide invaluable emotional support, practical assistance, and companionship throughout the hormone therapy journey. Their presence and understanding can offer comfort, encouragement, and a sense of belonging during times of uncertainty or difficulty.

- Healthcare Providers: Healthcare providers, including doctors, nurses, and other medical professionals, play a central role in providing clinical support, guidance, and expertise in hormone therapy. Establishing a trusting and collaborative relationship with healthcare providers can help individuals feel empowered, informed, and confident in their treatment decisions.

- Support Groups: Support groups, whether in-person or online, offer a unique opportunity for individuals undergoing hormone therapy to connect with others who share similar experiences, concerns, and challenges. Participating in support groups can provide a sense of camaraderie, validation, and mutual support, as well as access to valuable information, resources, and coping strategies.

- Community Organizations: Community organizations, advocacy groups, and non-profit organizations dedicated to hormone-related health issues can serve as valuable sources of information, education, and support for individuals undergoing hormone therapy. These organizations may offer educational materials, peer support programs, and advocacy efforts aimed at raising awareness and promoting access to care.

2. Benefits of Establishing a Support Network:

Establishing a network of support can offer numerous benefits for individuals undergoing hormone therapy, including:

- Emotional Support: Hormone therapy can be a challenging and emotionally demanding process, with potential physical, psychological, and social implications. Having a network of supportive individuals who understand and empathize with the challenges of hormone therapy can provide emotional validation, comfort, and reassurance during difficult times.

- Practical Assistance: Hormone therapy may require individuals to make lifestyle changes, adhere to treatment regimens, and navigate healthcare systems. Family members, friends, and healthcare providers can offer practical assistance, such as transportation to appointments, help with household tasks, or assistance in managing medication schedules, easing the burden of treatment and promoting adherence.

- Informational Guidance: Navigating the complexities of hormone therapy can be daunting, with a multitude of treatment options, side effects, and considerations to navigate. Healthcare providers, support groups, and community organizations can offer valuable informational guidance, answering questions, clarifying misconceptions, and providing evidence-based information to empower individuals to make informed decisions about their care.

- Sense of Belonging: Hormone therapy can sometimes lead to feelings of isolation, stigma, or alienation, particularly if individuals feel misunderstood or marginalized due to their health condition. Establishing a network of support can foster a sense of belonging, acceptance, and inclusion, providing individuals with a supportive community where they feel valued, understood, and accepted for who they are.

3. Building and Sustaining Support Networks:

Building and sustaining a network of support requires effort, intentionality, and reciprocity from all parties involved. Individuals undergoing hormone therapy can take proactive steps to nurture their support networks by:

- Communicating openly and honestly about their needs, concerns, and preferences with family members, friends, and healthcare providers.
- Seeking out support groups, community organizations, or online forums where they can connect with others who share similar experiences and challenges.
- Participating in educational events, workshops, or support group meetings to learn more about hormone therapy, coping strategies, and self-care practices.
- Offering support, encouragement, and understanding to others within their network, creating a culture of mutual support and reciprocity.

Healthcare providers can also play a vital role in facilitating the establishment and maintenance of support networks by:

- Providing patients with information, resources, and referrals to support groups or community organizations specializing in hormone-related health issues.
- Encouraging open communication and collaboration between patients, their families, and other members of their support network.
- Acknowledging and validating the emotional, social, and practical challenges of hormone therapy and offering compassionate support and guidance to patients and their loved ones.

In conclusion, establishing a network of support is essential for promoting well-being, resilience, and empowerment among individuals undergoing hormone therapy. By connecting with supportive individuals, communities, and resources, individuals can access the emotional, practical, and informational support they need to navigate the challenges of hormone therapy with confidence, resilience, and optimism. Whether through family, friends, healthcare providers, support groups, or community organizations, building and sustaining a network of support can make a profound difference in the treatment journey and contribute to enhanced quality of life and well-being.

The Value of Community: Creating Relationships That Promote Health and Well-Being

Communities are essential in forming our lives because they offer us a sense of belonging, support, and a common identity that improves our quality of life and enriches our experiences. Communities provide a vital network of connections and resources that can favorably impact a variety of elements of our lives, including physical health, mental health, and emotional resilience. These might range from neighborhoods and social circles to online forums and interest groups. We'll talk about the value of community and how fostering relationships may improve people's health and well-being both individually and as a group.

1. Social Cohesion and a Sense of Belonging:

The ideas of social support and belonging, which are crucial for fostering emotional well-being and resilience, are at the core of community. Being a part of a community helps people fight emotions of alienation, loneliness, and support by giving them a sense of connection, friendship, and support from one another. Communities provide a setting where people can feel appreciated, understood, and accepted for who they are, whether via shared experiences, common interests, or cultural links. This fosters a sense of identity and belonging that adds to overall pleasure and life satisfaction.

2. Promotion and Prevention of Health:

Communities provide environments that support healthy habits, lifestyles, and social norms, which are vital for improving health and preventing disease. Communities can encourage preventive screenings and vaccinations, raise awareness of important health issues, and give access to resources and services that support both physical and mental well-being through programs like wellness fairs, health education campaigns, and community health fairs. Communities may empower individuals to make educated decisions and take proactive measures to prioritize their own and their families' health by cultivating a culture of health and well-being.

3. Solidarity and Mutual Support:

Communities come together to support one another and those in need during difficult times, offering consolation, support, and useful aid. Communities have a unique ability to mobilize resources, coordinate relief efforts, and provide a helping hand to individuals and families facing problems, whether in response to natural catastrophes, economic troubles, or personal tragedies. Communities show the strength of group effort and the resiliency of the human spirit via deeds of kindness, generosity, and compassion. This creates a sense of togetherness and solidarity that fortifies links and increases resilience in the face of hardship.

4. Diversity and Cultural Enrichment:

By embracing variety, cultural history, and common customs that create a vibrant tapestry of experiences and viewpoints, communities enhance our lives. People can explore, respect, and learn about many cultures, customs, and traditions through cultural festivals, art events, and community get-togethers. This promotes intercultural understanding and appreciation. Communities may foster welcoming, inclusive settings that support human development, creativity, and teamwork by accepting variety and fostering inclusivity.

5. Collaborative Action and Social Capital:

Communities have social capital, which is characterized as the connections, resources, and networks that allow people to work together for the benefit of all. Communities may confront complicated social issues, push for positive change, and gather resources to deal with common problems by utilizing the power of social capital. Through community organizing, volunteerism, or grassroots action, people can use their combined power and influence to make a real difference and build a society that is more just, equal, and sustainable.

6. Mental Health and Well-Being Promotion:

Because they offer chances for meaningful participation, emotional support, and social contact, community connections are essential for fostering mental health and well-being. People can develop a sense of fulfillment, purpose, and belonging through friendships, social networks, and community activities. This promotes psychological resilience and emotional well-being. Positive interactions and the development of a sense of community can help people improve their mental health and acquire coping mechanisms that will make it easier for them to face obstacles in life with more hope and resilience.

In summary, the value of community in fostering resilience, happiness, and good health in both individuals and societies cannot be emphasized. Communities provide conditions that enhance social cohesion, mental health, and physical health by encouraging connections, belonging, and mutual support. These qualities improve our individual lives and increase our ability as a group to thrive. Communities have the ability to change lives, foster resilience, and pave the way for a better future for everybody through deeds of kindness, mutual support, or group efforts.

Talk about the importance of family and friends throughout menopause

The Value of Friends and Family During Menopause: Sharing the Experience

A woman's reproductive years come to an end with menopause, a major life shift that causes a variety of physical, emotional, and psychological changes. Family and friends' understanding and support are invaluable at this life-changing time, helping women deal with the difficulties and changes that come with menopause. The presence of loved ones can significantly impact how women experience and manage menopausal symptoms, from bringing companionship and understanding to practical assistance and emotional support. The significance of friends and family throughout menopause will be discussed, as well as how their assistance can enhance women's wellness at this time of life.

1. Emotional Assistance and Comprehension:

Hormonal shifts and bodily changes cause a rollercoaster of feelings that typically accompany menopause, including mood swings, impatience, anxiety, and melancholy. Family and friends' compassion and understanding can be a much-needed source of solace and confidence during this emotionally taxing period. Just knowing that loved ones are available to listen, lend a shoulder, and show unconditional support can go a long way toward making women feel less alone and more capable of handling the emotional highs and lows associated with menopause.

2. Help and Attention in Practice:

In addition to providing emotional support, family and friends may also help women with the day-to-day problems of menopause by providing care and practical assistance. The practical support of loved ones can lessen the stress of menopausal symptoms and free women to concentrate on their health and wellness. This assistance can take many forms, such as helping with domestic tasks, running errands, cooking meals, or providing transportation to medical appointments. Family and friends can show that they are committed to supporting women during this time of transition and making sure they are comfortable by offering a helping hand.

3. Friendship and Sympathy:

Menopause can occasionally feel like a lonely and alienating condition, especially for women who think they are experiencing it alone. In addition to delivering chances for social engagement, humor, and shared experiences that help combat feelings of loneliness and isolation, family and friends can offer much-needed camaraderie and companionship. The company of loved ones can uplift spirits, improve mood, and create a sense of connection and belonging through engagement in leisure activities, hobbies, and interests.

4. Advocacy and Empowerment:

In addition, friends and family can be extremely helpful in enabling women to take charge of their health and look for the right support and care during menopause. Loved ones may help women develop the confidence and self-advocacy skills they need to speak out, ask questions, and make decisions about their health and well-being by providing them with support, affirmation, and encouragement. Family and friends can also act as supporters and advocates for women by going to doctor's appointments with them, posing questions on their behalf, and offering moral support when speaking with medical professionals.

5. Information and Education:

Family and friends can help women better understand and become aware of menopause by educating them on the psychological, emotional, and physical changes that come with going through this stage of life. Loving relationships can help demystify menopause and encourage women to actively manage their health and wellness by exchanging personal experiences, having candid conversations about pertinent issues, and providing information about available coping mechanisms and treatment alternatives. Families and friends can also help women find trustworthy information sources to deepen their knowledge and comprehension of menopause, like healthcare practitioners, trustworthy websites, and support groups.

In conclusion, it is impossible to overestimate the value of friends and family throughout menopause. Their advocacy, companionship, practical help, and emotional support can make a big difference in women's resiliency and overall well-being during this time of change. Women who have good connections and encourage open communication can rely on their loved ones for support, direction, and empathy as they deal with the difficulties and transitions associated with menopause. Families and friends working together can foster an atmosphere that empowers menopausal women and supports their well-being.

Emphasize the value of shared experiences

Highlighting the Benefits of Shared Experiences: Creating Stronger Relationships and Promoting Development

Our relationships are woven together by shared experiences, which bind us to one another in deep and significant ways. Sharing life's moments, whether it be through happy events, difficult times, or just day-to-day experiences, helps to build relationships, develop empathy, and improve our comprehension of one another. We'll talk about the importance of shared experiences and how they enhance our sense of identity, personal development, and depth of relationships in this topic.

1. Creating Relationships and Trust:

Our relationships are based on shared experiences, which establish a foundation of understanding and promote a feeling of unity and connection. Our shared experiences, whether they involve going on adventures, overcoming obstacles, or commemorating significant occasions, help us to form memories that last a lifetime and transcend space and time. Our relationships are strengthened and our sense of belonging is enhanced when these shared memories serve as the cornerstone of intimacy, trust, and understanding.

2. Building Compassion and Empathy:

Sharing our experiences with others helps us understand their feelings, ideas, and viewpoints, which improves empathy and compassion in our relationships. Even for a short while, putting ourselves in another person's shoes helps us understand their perspective on the world and gain a deeper understanding of their particular struggles and experiences. Empathy fosters a sense of unity and reciprocal assistance, allowing us to provide consolation, comprehension, and motivation to individuals we hold dear during life's ups and downs.

3. Encouraging Individual Development and Adaptability:

Because they expose us to fresh viewpoints, concepts, and chances for education and self-discovery, shared experiences can accelerate personal development and resilience. The challenges we face through shared experiences—whether they include conquering barriers, battling anxieties, or embracing new experiences—provide a rich environment for development and transformation. We may discover the bravery and strength to step beyond our comfort zones, welcome change, and take advantage of life's growing chances by relying on one another for support and encouragement.

4. Building Relationships and Communication:

By offering a common language and framework for communication, shared experiences act as catalysts for deeper connections and meaningful interactions. Shared experiences provide a rich basis for meaningful conversation and connection, whether it's reminiscing about past adventures, reflecting on shared triumphs and struggles, or talking about common interests and hobbies. We improve our mutual understanding and fortify the ties of intimacy and trust in our relationships by opening up to one another about our thoughts, feelings, and experiences.

5. Building Traditions and Lasting Memories:

In addition to enhancing our lives and fostering a feeling of continuity and tradition in our families and relationships, shared experiences provide enduring memories. The memories we make via shared experiences become priceless treasures that we keep with us throughout our lives, whether they are holiday customs, yearly rituals, or impromptu excursions. We are woven together in a web of common experiences and beliefs by these cherished memories, which act as markers of our shared past.

In summary, the importance of shared experiences in our relationships and sense of identity in the world cannot be emphasized. Sharing life experiences, whether through joyous occasions, difficult times, or just day-to-day moments, fortifies relationships, encourages empathy, and expands our comprehension of one another. We may develop stronger bonds, encourage personal development, and make enduring memories that improve our lives and the lives of others we care about by embracing the power of shared experiences.

Promote pursuing treatment as a means of achieving emotional well-being.

Encouraging Therapy as a Route to Emotional Wellness: Enabling People to Give Their Mental Health First Priority

The significance of mental and emotional well-being for total wellness has gained attention in recent years. The stigma associated with getting treatment for mental health problems still exists, though, and keeps a lot of people from getting the care they require. Encouraging people to seek therapy is essential for achieving emotional well-being because it gives them the capacity to take charge of their mental health, ask for help, and start a path toward recovery and development. In this conversation, we'll look at the advantages of getting emotional wellness therapy as well as tactics for raising mental health awareness and increasing access to care.

1. Recognizing the Significance of Mental Well-Being:

Mental health is just as important to our entire welfare as physical health is in determining our thoughts, feelings, and actions. A variety of elements contribute to emotional well-being, such as resilience, self-worth, coping mechanisms, and the capacity to effectively handle stress and deal with life's obstacles. By recognizing the significance of mental health, we can foster a society that places a high value on emotional well-being, lessens the stigma associated with getting help, and motivates people to take proactive measures to take care of their mental health.

2. Finding Assistance and Materials:

To pursue treatment for emotional health, one must have access to resources and assistance that cater to their unique needs and concerns. This can include holistic approaches to mental health and wellness, pharmaceutical management, therapy, counseling, support groups, and self-help techniques. By providing people with the right tools and resources, we enable them to look into alternative healing options, learn coping mechanisms, and become resilient in the face of hardship.

3. Tackling Treatment-Related Barriers:

Even though getting treatment for emotional well-being is important, several obstacles might make it difficult to get care, such as stigma, lack of understanding, financial difficulties, and a shortage of mental health facilities. A multifaceted strategy is needed to address these obstacles, one that involves increasing access to affordable care, decreasing stigma, promoting culturally competent and inclusive mental health services, and increasing public awareness. We can make the healthcare system more accessible and helpful for everyone by pushing for legislative changes, boosting funding for mental health initiatives, and de-stigmatizing getting help.

4. Encouraging People to Ask for Help:

To empower people to seek treatment for their emotional well-being, it is important to create a welcoming, accepting environment where people feel comfortable talking about their mental health issues and asking for assistance when necessary. This could entail promoting self-care behaviors that put mental health and well-being first, sharing personal accounts of recovery and resilience, and de-stigmatizing seeking treatment through education and awareness campaigns. We can foster a culture that values and promotes mental health by promoting open communication, understanding, and compassion. This will enable people to seek treatment without worrying about prejudice or judgment.

5. Advancing Wholesome Well-Being:

Seeking therapy for emotional health is a component of a larger effort to achieve holistic wellness, which takes the mental, emotional, and spiritual aspects of health into account. The integration of mental health services into regular medical procedures and the advocacy of a comprehensive wellness approach can effectively tackle the interdependence of the mind, body, and spirit, thereby fostering resilience and general well-being. To enhance emotional balance and resilience, this may entail implementing mindfulness exercises, stress-reduction strategies, physical activity, and good lifestyle choices into everyday routines.

6. Honoring Development and Fortitude:

Seeking help for one's mental health is a brave and self-empowering decision that should be honored. We recognize people's bravery, tenacity, and resolve to overcome obstacles and succeed by recognizing their growth and resilience in their mental health journeys. This might be celebrating victories, highlighting life milestones, and offering people continuous support and motivation through the highs and lows of their mental health journey.

To sum up, encouraging therapy as a way to achieve emotional well-being is crucial to giving people the confidence to put their mental health first, ask for help, and start a path toward recovery and development. We can establish a culture that values and supports emotional well-being for everyone by recognizing the significance of mental health, providing access to resources and support, removing obstacles to treatment, empowering people to ask for help, encouraging holistic wellness, and applauding accomplishments and resilience. By working together, we can eliminate stigma, increase access to care, and advance a more accepting and encouraging mental health culture that enables people to lead happy, healthy lives.

Chapter 9

Accepting the Next Section

Taking the Next Step and Embracing Development and Change

Transitions are inevitable in life; they usher in new chapters in our individual and societal stories. Transitions offer chances for development, learning, and self-realization, whether they involve starting a new career, relocating to a new place, or entering a new relationship. It can be difficult to navigate change, though, as it requires us to let go of the known and bravely and resiliently embrace the unknown. We'll talk about the significance of accepting the next phase of our path and the transformational potential of embracing change in this conversation.

1. Accepting Change as a Growth Catalyst:

Life will inevitably involve change, which offers us chances for development, education, and self-discovery. Even though change can be unpleasant and painful, it also presents an opportunity to break free from ingrained habits, broaden our perspectives, and uncover untapped opportunities. We may use change's transforming potential to advance on our path of spiritual and personal development if we welcome it with an open heart and mind.

2. Leaving the Past Behind:

Letting go of the past, severing ties to the past, and opening ourselves up to the possibility of the future are frequently necessary steps in accepting the next. This can be a challenging process because we might experience melancholy, loss, or anxiety about the future. But when we let go of regrets, resentments, and attachments and instead acknowledge and honor our prior experiences, we make room for new experiences, relationships, and possibilities to arise.

3. Building Adaptability and Resilience:

Resilience and adaptability are necessary to embrace change as we negotiate the unknowns and difficulties that come with transitions. We can overcome challenges, recover from setbacks, and face adversity with bravery and tenacity when we possess resilience. We can handle change more easily and gracefully by building resilience via self-care routines, mindfulness, and constructive coping mechanisms. By doing so, we may have faith in our capacity to ride out life's storms and come out stronger on the other side.

4. Determining Purpose and Meaning:

Aligning our intentions and behaviors with our core beliefs, interests, and goals is a necessary part of accepting the next step. We may determine the course of our journey and make deliberate moves toward our objectives and aspirations by thinking back on what is important to us and what makes us happy and fulfilled. We may live truly and intentionally when we embrace change, whether that means choosing a new professional route, pursuing our artistic passions, or building meaningful relationships. This helps us to live by our innermost beliefs.

5. Seeking Advice and Assistance:

It can be difficult to navigate change, so it's critical to look for support and direction from people who have been there before or who can provide perspective and insights. Reaching out for help may bring us the inspiration, insight, and assurance we need to handle change with confidence and resilience. This support can come in the form of professional assistance from therapists or coaches, advice from mentors, or confiding in reliable friends.

6. Accepting the Self-Discovery Journey:

Accepting the next step involves embracing the process of self-realization and self-discovery as well as external changes. We have the chance to investigate our values, beliefs, and aspirations as we negotiate change, and we may discover buried strengths, passions, and abilities that have lain dormant within us. We can develop a greater sense of self-awareness, authenticity, and fulfillment by welcoming the journey of self-discovery with curiosity and openness. This will help us to match our lives with our true purpose and potential.

To sum up, taking the next step is a brave act that calls on us to welcome change with resiliency, openness, and faith in life as it unfolds. Transitions can be navigated with grace and confidence if we let go of the past, develop resilience, find meaning and purpose, seek support and guidance, and embrace the journey of self-discovery. This will enable us to embrace the unknown and build a future full of possibility, growth, and fulfillment.

Celebrating knowledge

Encourage women to embrace their experience and knowledge

Honoring Wisdom: Encouraging Women to Accept Their Experience and Intelligence

Knowledge is a potent instrument that people may use to overcome obstacles in life, make wise decisions, and bring about positive change in their own lives and the lives of others. Particularly women have accumulated a plethora of knowledge and wisdom through life experiences, personal development, and perseverance in the face of hardship. Through commemorating knowledge and urging women to cherish their distinct experiences and perspectives, we may enable them to acknowledge their value, appreciate their contributions, and reach their maximum potential. We'll talk about the value of honoring knowledge and how women may use their knowledge to make a positive difference in both their own lives and the lives of others.

1. Aware of the Worth of Life Experience:

Women's experiences have shaped perceptions, attitudes, and values in significant ways. They are a rich tapestry of struggles, victories, and lessons gained. Through overcoming cultural barriers and systemic injustices, women's lived experiences provide a unique prism through which to perceive the world and influence good change, ranging from navigating relationships and employment. By appreciating the significance of lived experience, we celebrate the resourcefulness, fortitude, and growth potential of women and enable them to confidently and proudly accept their journey.

2. Valuing the Diversity of Opinions:

Each woman's journey is distinct, molded by her own identity, culture, and heritage. By honoring the variety of viewpoints and voices within the women's community and realizing that every woman has unique experiences, insights, and skills to offer, we celebrate knowledge. Embracing this range of viewpoints encourages empathy, compassion, and unity among women from all walks of life, enriching our collective understanding of the world.

3. Adopting an Intergenerational Perspective:

The wisdom that women have passed down through the ages, across nations, and through traditions is one of the most precious sources of information. Younger women can benefit from the experiences and lessons of their elders by embracing intergenerational wisdom, and they can obtain insightful advice, mentorship, and guidance that will inform their own journeys. Similarly, elder women can find joy in imparting their knowledge and experience to the following generation, so creating a long-lasting legacy of inspiration and empowerment.

4. Encouraging Continuous Education:

Honoring the past is only one aspect of celebrating knowledge; another is encouraging a culture of continuous learning and development. Women are naturally lifelong learners; they are always looking for new ways to grow both personally and professionally, to broaden their horizons, and to learn new things. We enable women to take on new challenges, explore their hobbies, and pursue their goals with confidence and zeal by cultivating a love of learning and curiosity.

5. Encouraging Self-Belief and Self-Respect:

Celebrating knowledge also aims to enhance women's self-esteem and confidence by highlighting their contributions to society and intrinsic worth. By recognizing their accomplishments, experience, and skills, we encourage women to be confident in their own abilities and speak out for themselves in all spheres of life. This self-worth lays the groundwork for women to be empowered on a personal level, allowing them to speak up, follow their dreams, and push for improvements both inside and outside of their communities.

6. Establishing Areas for Exchange and Cooperation:

Celebrating knowledge entails setting up forums where women may exchange experiences, perspectives, and knowledge, encouraging cooperation, camaraderie, and support from one another. These spaces—whether they be community forums, women's circles, or mentorship programs—offer women the chance to interact, share knowledge, and work together on projects that further their common objectives. We can increase the effect of women's knowledge and build

a more inclusive and fair society by promoting a
culture of cooperation and group wisdom.

To sum up, valuing women's lived experiences,
welcoming a diversity of viewpoints, and promoting
a culture of lifelong learning and development are
all part of celebrating knowledge. We create a world
where women are empowered to thrive and
meaningfully contribute to their communities and
society at large by encouraging them to realize their
innate worth, respect their contributions, and share
their insights with others. Let's honor learning and
the remarkable women whose tenacity, courage,
and wisdom enhance our lives.

Change the focus from loss to development

Shifting the Attention from Destruction to Progress:
Accepting Development and Metamorphosis

Transitions characterize life's journey and offer
chances for development, education, and
self-discovery. Even while feelings of uncertainty
and loss are frequently associated with change, it
also creates opportunities for fresh experiences and
directions in life. We can welcome change as a
stimulus for individual and group development by

reorienting our attention from what we've lost to the possibilities for growth and transformation. We'll talk about how important it is to shift our attention from loss to development and how doing so can help us be more resilient and upbeat when navigating life's transitions.

1. Accepting Change as a Growth Catalyst:

Life is full of natural and inevitable change, which offers us chances for development, self-discovery, and transformation. Although changes can initially cause emotions of anxiety or loss, they also present an opportunity to reinvent oneself, investigate novel avenues, and welcome novel experiences. We can approach life's transitions with a sense of curiosity, openness, and excitement by reinterpreting change as a catalyst for progress and embracing the opportunities for personal growth and transformation that lie ahead.

2. Determining Significance and Objective in Shifts:

Transitions force us to consider our values, objectives, and goals, whether they be changes in our relationships, careers, or personal situations. Transitions may be transforming; by giving them meaning and purpose, we can make our behaviors

more in line with our innermost wishes and ideals.
Transitions offer rich opportunities for spiritual and
personal development, whether we're pursuing a
new passion, strengthening our relationships with
others, or setting out on a self-discovery trip.

3. Building Adaptability and Resilience:

To shift our attention from loss to progress, we
must learn to be resilient and adaptable to change.
Transitions can present opportunities to develop
inner strength, adaptability, and resourcefulness
even while they can also present difficulties and
setbacks. We may learn to handle life's ups and
downs with grace and resilience by accepting
change with an open mind and heart. We can
accomplish this by believing that we can overcome
hurdles and flourish in the face of adversity.

4. Investigating Novel Prospects and Opportunities:

A sense of opportunity and adventure are
frequently associated with transitions as we explore
new avenues for growth and experiences. By
accepting change as a chance for growth, we can
broaden our perspectives, get out of our comfort
zones, and discover new hobbies and interests. A
new career, a trip to a foreign place, or the

development of new relationships—transitions present countless opportunities for development and discovery.

5. Encouraging a Growth Mentality:

Developing a growth mindset is crucial to shifting the emphasis from loss to development because it enables us to see obstacles as chances for improvement. Setbacks can be viewed as instructive experiences that advance our professional and personal growth rather than as failures. To navigate life's transitions with confidence and tenacity, we can develop resilience, optimism, and a sense of agency by promoting a growth mindset.

6. Remembering Advancements and Turning Points:

Lastly, shifting the emphasis from loss to development entails acknowledging and appreciating our accomplishments along the path. Every stride we take ahead, whether it is by conquering challenges, accomplishing objectives, or hitting significant milestones, is evidence of our fortitude, bravery, and resolve. Recognizing and appreciating our accomplishments helps us maintain our optimism, confidence, and sense of self-worth as we go through life, which in turn propels us forward.

To sum up, accepting change as a driver for progress and transformation requires shifting the emphasis from loss to development. We may overcome life's obstacles with resiliency, optimism, and a sense of purpose if we reframe changes as chances for growth, exploration, and self-discovery. Accepting change as a necessary component of life's journey, let's approach changes with curiosity, openness, and excitement for what may be ahead.

Offer advice on how to have a meaningful life after menopause, including continuing therapy support

Getting By in Life After Menopause: Developing Purpose and Health

A woman's menopause signifies the end of an important phase in her life but also the beginning of fresh chances for development, fulfillment, and self-discovery. It's critical to investigate strategies for fostering well-being and meaning that are consistent with women's values, interests, and objectives as they move into this next stage of their lives. During this time, ongoing therapeutic support can be a tremendous help, offering direction, affirmation, and empowerment to women as they manage the mental, emotional, and physical changes that come with menopause. We'll cover tips on living a fulfilling life after menopause in this talk, stressing the value of ongoing therapeutic assistance.

1. Appreciate Self-Relationship and Research:

Women have the chance to pursue new passions, interests, and activities that make them happy and fulfilled after menopause. A sense of purpose and vitality can be found in experiencing new things, which can enhance life after menopause. Some examples of these experiences include taking up a new hobby, engaging in creative pursuits, or starting a self-discovery journey. A sense of surprise, enthusiasm, and curiosity about what lies ahead can be fostered in women by being open to new chances and welcoming change.

2. Give your physical and emotional well-being priority:

A satisfying life beyond menopause requires maintaining one's physical and mental well-being. Women can manage menopausal symptoms, sustain energy levels, and promote overall well-being with the support of regular exercise, a balanced diet, and enough sleep. Prioritizing self-care activities like stress reduction, mindfulness, and relaxation can also help to maintain emotional equilibrium and resilience during this time of change. Sustaining treatment can provide extra methods and resources for handling stress, adjusting to changes in life, and improving mental health.

3. Build Deeply Meaningful Connections:

A fulfilling life is built on meaningful connections, which offer companionship, support, and connection through difficult times. Women may discover that their social networks change after menopause, offering them fresh chances to build new connections and strengthen current ones. Women navigating the ups and downs of life after menopause can find support, purpose, and a sense of belonging by cultivating meaningful relationships with friends, family, and community members.

4. Take Part in Growth and Lifelong Learning:

Beyond menopause, retaining energy and fulfillment in life requires lifelong study and personal development. Whether it takes the form of going to classes, attending seminars and workshops, or just learning about new concepts and viewpoints, intellectual and personal development may pique curiosity, kindle enthusiasm, and provide a feeling of achievement and purpose. Sustained therapy support can offer direction and inspiration to women as they delve into their passions, establish objectives, and surmount barriers to their own development and satisfaction.

5. Discover Purpose and Meaning in Serving and Giving:

After menopause, a deep feeling of purpose and fulfillment can be found in helping others and changing the world for the better. Giving back to their communities and improving the lives of others can provide women a sense of purpose and fulfillment, whether through volunteer work, mentoring, or supporting charities that share their values. Women who receive ongoing therapeutic support can better understand their beliefs, passions, and significant ways to contribute to society.

6. Maintain Contact with Counseling Assistance:

Support from ongoing treatment can be a great tool for women adjusting to life beyond menopause. Women can examine their thoughts, process life changes, and create coping mechanisms for handling menopausal symptoms and other difficulties in a safe and encouraging environment with the help of therapists. During this phase of transition, women may find themselves navigating the complexity of relationships, professional changes, and personal growth. In these situations, therapy can provide advice and validation. Women who continue to engage in treatment can obtain the resources, understanding, and encouragement needed to develop a purposeful and happy postmenopausal life.

To sum up, the postmenopausal era presents women with a period of change, development, and a chance to discover novel avenues, foster significant connections, and derive satisfaction from their interests and endeavors. Sustaining therapy may be a tremendous source of empowerment, validation, and assistance for women navigating the emotional, psychological, and physical changes that come with this transforming time. Women can design a meaningful, purposeful, and fulfilling life after

menopause by embracing self-discovery, putting
their well-being first, building meaningful
relationships, learning and growing throughout life,
finding meaning in service and contribution, and
maintaining contact with therapy support.